REVEALING GOD'S DESIGN FOR AGING, FAMILY, AND HOW WE LIVE

A Biblical, Cultural, and Practical View of Aging

7/24/22

Dorothy!

I'm so glad you are an important part of RGU & for sharing your life with us!

Blessings!

Bob

Bob Benson

ISBN 978-1-63885-870-6 (Paperback)
ISBN 978-1-63885-871-3 (Digital)

Covenant Books
11661 Hwy 707
Murrells Inlet, SC 29576
www.covenantbooks.com

To the mentors who inspired me to labor,
to the elders who taught me to listen,
to Nina and our children, who encourage me to laugh, and
to Jesus, who stirs me to love.

CONTENTS

INTRODUCTION

I suppose it's like the ticking crocodile, isn't it?
Time is chasing after all of us.
—J.M. Barrie, Peter Pan

In J. M. Barrie's original 1904 play, *Peter Pan*, the Lost Boys were spirited to Neverland because they fell out of their strollers and remained unclaimed for seven days. Neverland would be an ideal existence with many adventures led by Peter Pan. However, they could remain part of the Lost Boys only so long as they believed in the magic. When they no longer believed, they returned to England where they would grow up. Wendy, the only girl involved (according to Pan, girls were too smart to fall out of their baby buggies), grew up, married, and had a daughter who looked for Pan.

There is a sadness in Peter Pan: the loss of youth and innocence. We recognize it because we, too, grew up, and whatever innocence we might have had was lost along the way—some before others. Many of us perceive aging similarly. We somehow grow into our teens and young adulthood with energy and drive. At that time, becoming aged is a far-off mystical thing—it happens but is lost in the mist and not much thought is given to it.

Until we begin to age, we hear the Peter Pans of our culture telling us that youth, strength, and beauty are foremost in our culture. Hold on to youth; take steps to stay forever young. Almost anywhere we look, we find examples of people drawn by the power of our culture's enamor with youth. Plenty of resources are telling us about aging—the preservation of self—but many of them point to how to retain youth, as though it is all that aging is about.

7

Peter Pan is sad in another sense. Eternal youth has its allure but misses the gifts that come only from aging and the challenges to get there. Peter Pan cannot imagine life beyond all play and adventures. Peter Pan, and perhaps we, cannot fathom that aging endows us with precious gifts. God's design for our aging is an unpredictable blessing requiring an occasional nerve-wracking walk of faith but something to look forward to as well. There be gifts!

With about ten thousand people turning sixty-five every day in the US, the vision of our culture still seems driven to retain youth. Advertisements and media blitzes show older people actively engaged in activities that at one time were almost unthinkable for older people. A positive, healthy attitude about aging is applaudable. Huge numbers of articles, books, blogs, and podcasts extol the latest research and how to live well until we die. These things have their place, and they can be helpful in many ways. What if we stopped to think about how those attitudes cultivated in society are just that: attitudes driven by a distinct worldview. How do these ideas on aging sync with a Christian worldview? Should we take our culture's ideals and consider them biblical just because this is America? Is it even possible to think about aging from God's perspective?

This is not a book about how to age well, or how to retain youthful vigor, or even about ageism. Rather, it is an exploration of aging from a biblical perspective in which God sheds light on his thoughts of our aging. This work intends to help reveal your attitudes and biases to some degree and to shed light on some of the key issues of aging in the home, families, and culture relative to Scripture. It compares what many readers experience and think with how God communicates about elders and the frail. How his love never fails.

Aging is God's design for us. Chapter 1 searches how Scripture describes the nature of time and aging itself—why we age, for instance. Following that important background, this book explores six aspects of aging that the Scriptures address. Chapter 2 discusses how the Bible offers a distinct perspective of aging based on God's design. It briefly discusses our cultural perspectives of life expectancy and aging. It contrasts those perspectives with the elements God put into place that benefit the aging (of whom a disproportionate number are poor). Reviewing the social structures God established through Israel's laws demonstrates his exercise of compassion and provision for older people. The chapter ends by exploring the respectful use of words the writers of Scripture used to describe or address elders.

The third chapter considers how God provides special gifts to the aging. In our culture, we normally do not look at the aging process as a time of special gifting and growth. This chapter reviews several gifts that come through aging and how they might affect the elder and those around her or him. Some of the gifts are obvious, such as gaining experience over the years and the possibility of knowing God better or becoming wise. Other gifts, such as not feeling our age or how our emotions may be affected by our years, may be less familiar to the reader. Recognizing and leveraging the gifts is an important tool in understanding and relating to elders while helping them to succeed in their purposes of loving God and enjoying Him forever.

Building on the earlier chapters, chapter 4 uses a biblical lens to shift to advocacy. Prime examples found in Scripture inform us about what it means to advocate for our aging families. If a friend, family, or professional is not seen as an advocate, any approach for supporting an aging person will be more difficult. Being seen as a trusted advocate is essential to working successfully with elders.

The following chapters transition to explore physical, financial, relational, mental, spiritual, and emotional aspects as we relate to our own aging as well as those aging around us.

Chapter 5 identifies some of the transitions occurring in the aging and how that can affect personal and family life. The Scriptures offer perspectives that may help the readers put aging into the greater context of life and family. The chapter explores the continuous transition we have in life and that the aging often experience multiple types of chronic illnesses. It reveals some of the more common causes of unnecessary death and how to identify issues and trends before they become problematic.

Chapter 6 discusses issues regarding money, noting that many people often imply that the measure of life may be the size of a portfolio or bank balance. This chapter reviews some aspects of aging and money from a few perspectives. While drawing on Scripture as a guide, it discusses finances and the use of money in aging from several moral and ethical angles. After all, what benefit is there in gaining the whole world yet losing the soul?

Chapter 7 focuses on how aging family members might create unique challenges and problems while living in the homes of their adult children. This chapter explores what the Scriptures teach on caring for family members in our homes and how God's Word can inform discussions in difficult family dynamics with both believers and unbelievers. The intent is not to answer the specific issues in detail but to provide New and Old Testament frameworks from which elder care can be viewed relative to the family.

Finally, chapter 8 summarizes the discussion of these parts of Scripture, how we might consider the wisdom of God's design of aging, and how we might look forward to and enjoy aging as a gift He bestows.

This book is not a comprehensive review of aging and its challenges. I selected the topics based on my observations of families and elders and identifying some of the common roadblocks they experience. I am not a clinician, social worker, researcher, or biblical scholar. Nothing within this should be taken as medical advice or the final word in understanding Scripture. However, I have over forty years of experience working with elders and their families while managing long-term health and housing services in independent living, assisted living, adult day service, home health, hospice, durable medical equipment, and nursing homes in multiple states. Observation and conflict resolution through much prayer and many mistakes form the basis of my opinions and insights.

On the journey of this writing, I hope that you will find illumination, insight, and support in your perspective on aging and working with the aging. It is my prayer that in this work, the Scriptures may provide some guidance, strength, and comfort as we age.

After all, time is like a ticking crocodile chasing after us.

To God be the glory.

Bob Benson
May 2021

1

Purpose in Aging

About thirty-five people had gathered in a seminar room. All the participants appeared to be in their twenties or thirties—young, compared with the instructor. The subject matter was to study the life stages of people and understand their various functions and needs through life. The seminar leader had all the participants in the room close their eyes and rest quietly while she read a narrative.

"Picture the person I am describing. He is generally happy, though he cannot communicate well. He needs help with about everything in life. Food gets all over his face every time he eats; he cannot hold a spoon and dribbles when using a cup. He sleeps a lot, even though he frequently wakes at night, and he needs help with his physical needs—bathing, dressing, and changing after accidents. He is not able to walk well, so he needs help to move from place to place. When cold, he gets a little cranky, and he flails around when things do not go as he thinks they should. He has a wonderful smile and twinkling eyes and a small thin tuft of hair around the crown of his head.

"Now that you have heard his description, where would you expect to find him today?"

The participants gave a variety of answers, suggesting a nursing home, assisted living center, or hospital. Someone proposed that, perhaps, he might be in hospice. Finally, the room turned silent.

"Let me show you a picture of him," the presenter said as she turned to the large screen at the room's front. On it was an eight-foot-wide image of a smiling baby reaching for the camera. "Meet my six-month-old grandson, Kyle."

What picture came to your mind as you read the story above? If in your mind you saw a frail older person, you would not be alone. It is common for people to picture the aged as frail, tottering, forgetful, and so many other negative things. It is true that some older people are frail, but the greater majority are not. Perhaps we do not think of the aging in terms of courage, strength, and experience because that description depicts aging people we do not recognize. Older women sometimes say that the problem with wrinkles and gray hair is that it renders them invisible. While this may happen to most older people at times, people of different racial or ethnic backgrounds commonly experience this, no matter their age. Invisible people are not ignored; they are nonexistent, not requiring attention.

Is this how you view aging? Have you observed that the elderly are not noticed until they cause problems at the grocery store or when they drive slowly in front of you? How about your aging? Have you decided not to age and do as a television ad once said, "Not age gracefully but fight it the whole way"? Why is it that the person staring back at us in the bathroom mirror looks so much older than the way we feel? Do our outward bodies tell a story that does not feel like us?

Imagine if we were rewarded for every new line we find on our faces, and even encouraging notice from others when each line becomes a deep crease. What if every blotch and blip on our faces and hands created a small celebration—an outward exhibition of inward growth that makes us more uniquely ourselves each passing day? What if every painful moment meant something and was a metamorphosis into the new better self? What if every perceived physical loss helped us turn to God rather than an attempt to restore youth and vigor?

In our thoughts of meaning and purpose, we usually do not ponder the purposes and gifts of the aging process. While other cultures seem to revere aged people, our "enlightened," postmodern

America considers that being young and strong is the way to "live the dream," and anything else is less than relevant. Every year Americans spend billions of dollars to look younger, yet ironically, they cannot outlive aging. The questions we must answer are these:

- Did God design us to age?
- What might be God's purpose and gifts that we experience because of aging?
- Is becoming aged an honorable state?

Over three thousand years ago, the teacher in Ecclesiastes discovered the importance of purpose while helping us to focus on the right purpose. After all, wisdom and knowledge had been searched, he concluded the following:

> Now all has been heard;
> Here is the conclusion of the matter:
> Fear God and keep his commandments
> For this is the duty of all mankind.
> For God will bring every deed into judgement,
> Including every hidden thing,
> Whether it is good or evil. (Eccles. 12:13–14)

Or the wisdom of James:

> Why, you do not even know what will happen
>   tomorrow.
> What is your life?
> You are a mist that appears for a little while and
>   then vanishes. (James 4:14)

The Scriptures teach us to number our days and consider that life is like a mist in the morning, gone like the morning's dew when the sun shines hotly. In that mist, our numbered days on earth, we change over time and our bodies age. Is aging without a point? Are we just to look at life and consider our best days were the ones in our twenties and thirties? Is there a purpose in aging, or is the corruption brought into the world through sin the cause of aging? Does God give us things to look forward to as we age? Are there gifts he provides expressly to those over sixty? This book attempts to explore aspects of aging and relationships in aging from the Scripture's viewpoint.

We are provided with an inherent purpose for our lives and aging. This purpose is from an intimate, knowledgeable, well-resourced God, who established and loves us individually and completely. A loving God would not create a person he loves without reason. The evidence for that is specifically seen in the Scriptures—some details of that are coming here, but first we need to consider our purpose and the nature of time.

If our sole purpose is to reproduce ourselves, then after our children are born and raised, we should die like insects after mating. God clearly had more in mind for us than just preserving our species. Think about it, the life lifespan of people recorded in Genesis is hundreds of years. And even in our comparatively short lifetimes, many of the enjoyments, discoveries, and talents we find only come after living many years. Some of these things that grow in time are to love and nurture grandchildren, enjoy all of nature, marvel at the array of colors in our world, experience using all of our senses, and create friendships even late in life. There are many reasons for our entire lives to be numbered in many years. Some aspects of life are reserved for later in life, and some purposes are simply for God's pleasure. Considering all in nature that envelops us, God must delight in creating and making that creation (us and our lives) meaningful, starting in our youth and carrying through all of our days. God made us for a purpose that may be discovered or become clear only in age. But did this loving God design us to get old?

Are We Intended to Age?

"The glory of young men is their strength, gray hair the splendor of the old" (Prov. 20:29).

To answer this question, it helps to start at the Bible's beginning, looking at the sequence of creation. In Genesis 1, from before the first moments in time, God was. In Genesis 1:3–5, light and darkness were created, denoting a period defined as a "day." In God's plan, time is so vital, it warranted one-half of the first six verses of the Bible, immediately after God identified himself. The idea of time is so foundational that the idea of not having time is incomprehensible to us. Describing a time when there was no time is like trying to describe color to a person blind from birth. God made time a foundational principle of the universe; therefore, time, however we measure it, is essential.

After creating time, God designed a physical environment comprised of all things necessary for our survival. As the Master Architect, God created then personally certified that each step was good in the broadest possible interpretation. At the very end of the creation period, God inspected it one final time and declared it was "very good."

God shaped dust into human form and breathed his Spirit into it, creating man in his own image. Scripture uniquely highlights God's intimate cradling of Adam in his own image. God formed us then declared we were "very good." He made us in his image, matchless in creation, and gave us a particular blessing of a spoken role and purpose—unlike all other creatures. So God created time, place, and gave humans a beginning, a specific starting point in history, and a function in creation. Like the first man and woman, you and I did not preexist but were also placed into our time and in his creation.

God exclusively blessed Adam and Eve in ways that differentiated them from all of creation. In Genesis 1:28, God said, "Be fruitful and increase in number; fill the earth and subdue it. Rule over the fish of the sea and birds of the air and over every living creature that moves on the ground." The original Hebrew phrase rendered "be fruitful and increase in number" can be translated in either a narrow or broad sense. The narrow understanding is that Adam and Eve were to reproduce themselves and fill the earth with people. The broader interpretation is that man and woman should participate in many activities that bear fruit (i.e., create, husband, or make things to the glory of God), and that in each activity, an appropriate increase should be sought. In the strict context of filling the earth, our understanding of the narrow translation is more common—increase in number. Both interpretations make sense. God is creative and active and is in the process of doing things; therefore, it follows that humans created in his image should have a similar purpose of creating and bearing fruit (an increase) of some meaningful kind.

Because Adam and Eve were created subject to time and told to create an increase (in whatever sense), it implies that God expected them to have a future and an impact on the creation. And where there is both a point in time when life begins and expected future experiences, it means there will be aging. I am not speaking of negative effects of that aging; just that it is reasonable to think that since God gives us a beginning and a future with purpose, we were intended to age.

I realize it took many words to get us to what we already know: we get older with each moment, and we mark that aging by counting the days lived. It is essential to understand that aging is God's idea, planned in the original creation; blessed with the purpose to be fruitful; and commanded to multiply, subdue, and rule the creation. Knowing that we were designed to age forces us to consider our specific perspective of aging. Aging, in and of itself, is by God's design. Aging is not our enemy.

If God described our aging design as "very good," then why do we dislike aging so much? Is it that we know deep in our souls that each breath we take gives us life but is one closer to our last breath? Is it because we resent that He lives forever but we do not? Is it just our nature of sin underscored by pride or envy?

Not all of us hold a grudge against aging. My wife asked our grown children about some of their memories of Christmas and the holidays. One responded that she had to go to bed before the older kids (she had positive things to say too). When another of our children was young, we allowed him to stay up until midnight on New Year's Eve. His analysis of the night was, "So this is what the big guys do!" What child does not wish to be older to watch a movie, drive a car, stay up until midnight, or whatever? Teenagers, and even people in their twenties, often think of aging only in the context of either helping their parents deal with technology or when they get behind a slow, white-headed driver a tad taller than the steering wheel. It seems we think first of aging when our grandparents seem so old or it dawns on us that we or our parents are different as they age. Eventually, aging becomes personal—the day we realize we cannot run as fast, stay up so late, or the mirror no longer befriends us. Why is this a problem?

Pundits (or comedians) might say that aging gives us glimpses of our mortality (or in my case, it is more like a glimpse of my grandfather looking back at me in the mirror). There is a subtlety that disturbs us. For our first twenty-five or thirty years, we experience few blemishes, thinning hair, loosening and wrinkling of the skin, or loss of stamina, and everything on us generally works. Yet that first gray hair or the shadow of a wrinkle shocks us. And though this is unsettling, we explain it as if it is just part of "getting old." For some reason, we think these things should not or cannot be happening to us. We seem surprised and then subtly grieve the losses we feel in our aging. This is even more powerful if we are diagnosed with a serious illness or have a friend who has an illness or disease. It is not fair, and it does not feel right, for us to experience these things anyway. But if our design is "very good," what is making this happen? Was there a mistake? Were we created with planned obsolescence? If so, God made some grave mistakes.

Since God created the concept of aging and said it was "good," then to say that our experience of frailty is "normal aging" is not normal at all. It was not in the original design. And that design was not flawed; it was "very good." "Then Abraham breathed his last and died at a good old age, an old man and full of years; and he was gathered to his people" (Gen. 25:8).

A physician once said that we all have cancer in our bodies, but our immune systems keep it at bay. Another physician once told me that if all men live long enough, they will eventually deal with prostate cancer. True or not, these statements illustrate a point. Within each of us resides elements of corruption. The physical evidence is seen when our bodies attack themselves or fail to launch a defense against an external source. Microbes and viruses like Ebola, Marburg, and COVID-19 can take over our bodies and destroy us without the agent of disease making a moral decision or having a single thought. Other evidence of our corruption might be seen in the actions of people taking advantage of or attacking others physically or verbally. We must admit that this corruption is part of our daily experience in one way or another, the corruption resides within each of us, and the corruption is rampant, affecting everything and all we are, including our aging bodies.

Clearly, then, we carry the seeds of corruption and death within our bodies. And it should be no surprise to us that the physical corruption, though always present, often becomes more greatly expressed the closer we get to one hundred twenty years. Not all people equally experience corruption's negative effects. We know some people live longer and have better health and life experiences than others. Inconsistencies between people's later life experiences increase our angst over the unfairness of the aging process, camouflaging the fact that our corrupted bodies and minds entice many to blame God for his "apparent" failures. The irony is that we are the ones who are corrupted, even brought on the corruption, not God. Aging itself is not sin or evil, but we are subject to the effect of our physical (and moral) corruption taking its toll on our bodies. As the apostle Paul wrote, the sting of death is sin (1 Cor. 15:56).

We have choices in living, and the decisions for good or bad relative to maintaining our physical bodies do have an impact. With good choices, some actions may minimize or delay many of the physical effects of the corruption. But regardless of our choices, we will all surrender to gravity and time. Because of the corruption both within and outside of us, as we move through time, we will experience various difficult issues. God recognized those challenges and spoke to us about them in the Scriptures, both in the Old and New Testaments.

Application

Our life experience in aging is not a story of birth, taxes, and then our bodies sag and die. Instead, we are thoughtfully, specifically, and beautifully designed for meaningful purpose and activity: to share in the creative efforts of our Creator's life to impact others within the realm of our influence. This implies that living purposefully has no age limit. Regardless of age, socioeconomic status, or ethnicity, each person has intrinsic value and contributions to make. We likely will experience at least some decline in abilities as we age—I may not run as fast, or I may think more slowly than I once did—but research is now revealing that many of our losses are lifestyle issues and not the results of aging (e.g., if you lay in bed long enough, you will lose strength regardless of your age. Period). It is ironic how corruption can take advantage of our bad habits, which we tend to blame on others or God.

We must think about our perspectives of aging and the impact of the corruption implicit within our bodies over a lifetime. What do we believe about aging? Is it an enemy, or is it a motivator to maximize the positive impact we can make on life? Also, observe the aging people around us. Do we believe that they, too, have a purpose and an impact on us? What can we do to encourage and even help reignite one another to meaningful engagement and purposeful living? Reconnecting people with purpose can provide sustainable motivation for each of us to relate more deeply to one another and God.

Takeaway Thoughts

1. A thoughtful Creator has made each of us for a purpose.
2. Experiencing age is part of our design, and the Creator determined that it was good and blessed it.
3. The negative effects found in aging are from the nature of corruption within us (not necessarily just from corrupt acts).
4. We might be able to minimize or delay some of the results of the corruption through good choices.
5. The result of the good choices may be more days to live purposefully, or it may simply give us better days in which we can live our purpose more easily.
6. Consider:
   a. How can living each day looking for an "increase" in others' lives be a sustainable motivator?

b.   How powerful is connecting our individual purpose to the truth that each of us was thoughtfully, intimately designed by a loving God?

Questions for Consideration

Chapter 1 claims that our general purpose was planned for us by an intelligent, thoughtful designer God. Look up Psalm 57:2 (written before David was became king) and compare what he says about his purpose with his language in Psalm 138:8, written near the end of his life.

In the context of Acts 13, the apostle Paul argues that Jesus is the living Messiah. He quotes Psalm 16, where David says, "You will not abandon me to the grave, nor will you let your Holy One see decay." His point is that the psalmist prophesies about the Messiah's resurrection. Look closely at what Paul says in verse 36: "For when David had served God's purpose in his own generation, he fell asleep."

1.   Do these verses relate just to David's purpose? If not, how might they apply to you?
2.   Is it true or false that we have a general, designed purpose and a more specific purpose laid out by God? Explain your answer.
3.   In Psalm 57:2, David says that it is "God who fulfills His purpose for me." In what ways does that apply to you?
4.   What is your role and responsibility in fulfilling that purpose?
5.   After reading Luke 7:30, consider how it may apply to God's fulfilling his (specific) purpose in you.

2

Perspective of Aging

The YouTube video is grainy. It has good sound but poor resolution. It is a short video three teenage boys were making with a budget camera. Two of the boys were trying to do difficult skateboard moves on a suburban sidewalk. The third was working to get the best action angles on the camera. Their lighthearted banter was interrupted by screeching tires and a blasting car horn. With the camera still on, the boys turned to the commotion and captured the scene. A new sleek black convertible with its top down was stopped at the corner. A middle-aged male driver had pulled his car within inches of an older woman's left leg and was glaring over aviator sunglasses at her. Wearing a long black coat and holding a shopping bag, the older woman appeared to be asleep in the middle of the crosswalk. The driver raced the car engine and leaned hard on the horn. The woman startled awake. She shuffled a step or two as the driver raced the engine again and blared the horn. Without a glance, she swung her shopping bag around and hit the car's front bumper near the head-light. There was a loud pop; white dust blasted into the air as the car's air bag exploded, shocking the driver, and knocking his glasses askew. Not turning her head, the woman slowly shambled out of the camera frame without a losing step. The three boys laughed as the stunned driver sat with his convertible idling in the empty crosswalk.

It is hard to imagine this scene anywhere other than an American suburb. A muscle car and an impatient power-tie-wearing driver confronting a sleeping older woman. The video illustrates key elements of our postmodern era and how we perceive older people. As we age, we see ourselves as retaining vibrancy and relevance while many others perceive the oldest of the old as existing only on the margins of society, out of touch and irrelevant. This perception is so rampant that the news media do not grasp the irony of their reports of story after story about the mistreatment of elders while advertisements in the same media revere the cultural obsession with youth.

Other cultures seem to value the aged more than we do in the United States. A high school Chinese exchange student recently observed that their culture values older people. "They possess wisdom and experience. Why wouldn't we want to hear what the aged have to say?" Many segments of the Native American culture also believe the matriarchs and patriarchs are invaluable to the family and community. Some historians may argue that a hundred years ago, even the American settlers held older people in great esteem.

Many Americans believe that, back in bygone days, the average life span was only forty or fifty years, and anyone older than that was a rare commodity. The facts are that in 1900, once people passed safely to the age of sixty-five, their life expectancy was the same as sixty-five and older people in the year 2000. The data suggest that over the last century, life expectancy has not greatly increased for men or women who reach the age of sixty-five.[1] The average extension of life is only three to five years.

It is important to consider how long people lived once they made it to the age of sixty-five. The reason for the difference between life expectancy at birth in the US in 1900 versus the year 2000 is that twentieth-century health-care breakthroughs most benefited children before the age of five years. The nation's death rate for children was high at the beginning of the twentieth century. During the last century, public health sanitation and disease control and treatment advanced rapidly, most benefiting the young, vulnerable populations. This work greatly diminished infant mortality and childhood disease. And compared with the year 1900, many more children lived into adulthood in 2000.

The long-term effect on the US population is not that older people are living a great deal longer than they did a century ago, but that more people made it past childhood and now are living into their seventies and eighties. The other part of the equation is that the US birth rate has declined, so the number of older people is growing relative to the younger population. On a percentage basis, there are more older people now than a hundred years ago, and on average, they are living only several years longer than their grandparents did. The reason the sixty-five-plus age group is living longer is likely due to better nutrition, exercise, and health care throughout their lives, from birth to end of life.

The first baby boomer (post-World War II) turned sixty-five on January 1, 2011, and about ten thousand boomers reach that milestone *each day*. Based on lifestyle changes, education, and continuing advances in medicine, many experts anticipate the life expectancy for those who reach sixty-five today will increase at a faster rate now that the boomers (born between 1946 and 1964) are impacting the data. Research shows that how we live our lives over the years affects both our longevity and our quality of life during our later years. "How long your parents lived does not necessarily affect how long you will live. Instead, it is how you live your life that determines how old you will get."[2]

Compared with a hundred or even fifty years ago, a greater percentage of the US population is older today, and there are greater numbers of older people as well. The irony in these statistics is that while the population's average age is increasing, intense focus on retaining or recapturing our youth is likewise increasing. Advertisements unabashedly reference turning back the clock; feeling young; people are not really aging, they just have different numbers on their lab tests, and using this prescription will return them to "normal." There is a dark side to America's infatuation with remaining young. Aging bodies cannot sustain years of maltreatment or poor nutrition without consequence. Our bodies themselves belie the advertisers' claims. And there is a real sense of discrimination against the older person.

Too many older Americans continue to face
discrimination based on persistent stereotypes
and outdated assumptions about age and work.

> Age discrimination is legally wrong and has been
> since the ADEA took effect five decades ago.
> But it remains too common and too accepted in
> today's workplace. While attitudes about older
> workers, their abilities, and age discrimination
> have improved somewhat over the past 50 years,
> much more can and should be done to make age
> discrimination less prevalent and less accepted.[3]

Disregard or diminution of the aging is common in the country, and the oldest of the old are relegated to social invisibility in many communities, particularly if they are from a minority ethnicity or creed.

The Scripture's View on Aging

Is gray hair our splendor, as it says in Proverbs 20:29? Given the American cultural view of aging, let us turn to learn how the Scriptures speak of and perceive older people.

In a brief review, the first chapter demonstrated the perspective of the Scriptures. God designed us to age, and it was good, though we are subject to the spiritual and physical corruption caused by sin. Physical decline, health issues, and other negative experiences as we age are results of the corruption, of which we can influence some by our lifestyle choices and modern medicine. Ultimately though, unless the Lord returns first, we should expect the sting of death around us and within us. This inevitable end is difficult to face but is the natural and logical consequence of our fallen nature. Still, the teacher in Ecclesiastes 7:2 and 4 says, "It is better to go to a house of mourning than to go to a house of feasting, for death is the destiny of every man; the living should take this to heart... The heart of the wise is in the house of mourning, but the heart of fools is in the house of pleasure." While mortality is unpleasant, it does make us consider our days and God's purpose for us. According to the teacher, this is wisdom. In other words, our Creator God, in his wisdom, uses even death, which was meant for our ill, to call our attention to our complete corruption and desperate need for a relationship with him.

God's perspective is "I take no pleasure in the death of anyone, declares the Sovereign LORD. Repent and live!" (Ezek. 18:32). It makes sense that since he created us in his image, he would find death incongruent with the original design. And because he is all-knowing, the great corruption did not surprise or stymie him. His all-loving and all-powerful nature compel him to invite his creation to return to him despite the sting of sin. And he made a way through his love.

A Comment on God's Love

To know that love is true, it must be tested. True love is not self-serving and cannot compel the recipient to love in return. The first test of God's love, then, is asking, does he force us to love him, or does he invite us into his love? In authentic love, the object of love must be able to choose to respond to God's love. Authentic love, then, requires an element of risk for the one who loves. God loves each of us deeply and personally but will not compel us to love him in return. He loves us first, inviting and wooing us into a relationship with him. As the prophet wrote, "You will seek me and find me when you seek for me with all your heart" (Jer. 29:13).

A corollary test of genuine love is, how does the one who loves respond when love is not reciprocated? In nonreciprocated love, the one who loves experiences disappointment but cannot stop loving and inviting relationship. Throughout Scripture, God calls people to decide whether to follow him. Joshua called out to Israel, "Choose for yourselves whom you will serve" (Josh. 24:15). Jesus himself confirmed God's love offer to all people in John 3:16. "For God so loved the world that He gave His one and only Son, that whoever believes in him should have eternal life." In answer to the first test of love, God calls us to respond to him. God's love passes the second part of the test in Ezekiel 18:23 when he says, "'Do I take any pleasure in the death of the wicked?' declares the Sovereign LORD. 'Rather, am I not pleased when they turn from their ways and live?'"

While God's love is everlasting and true, it does have a boundary. God made one pathway through the strict requirements of his love, holiness, and justice. And the cost to create that pathway was the highest imaginable to God. The time of God's favor is now, say the Scriptures, while we yet live. Today is the time of entering God's favor and rest forever. Once in the grave, we can no longer access the way to God's love. Jesus taught a parable of the wedding feast. All were invited to come, but when they had arrived, the doors were closed, and those who refused to come were destroyed (Matt. 22:7). Exactly why God's love has the boundary to be available as a choice for us only while we live is not made clear in Scripture. However, choosing not to love the One who makes his love for us clear each day equates to rejection. Does love cease when spurned for a lifetime? Perhaps not, but consequences from a life of rejection do make sense to our worldly minds. The pathway's gate to God's love and favor is accessible only while we live on earth; the gate closes at our death, never to reopen for us.

Evidence of the incontrovertible fact of God's love for the aged (in promise and action) is throughout the Scriptures, revealing God's view of the aging. Some of the first people to recognize the Messiah were advanced in years. God blessed childless and aged Zacharia and Elizabeth with a son, John the Baptist, to announce the coming of the Messiah. Elizabeth felt the unborn baby jump in her womb at Jesus's mother's voice. When Joseph and Mary presented Jesus to the aged Simeon in the temple, he prophesied that the baby Jesus would be a light to the gentiles and the glory of Israel. Eighty-four-year-old Anna came upon Jesus's parents during Simeon's prophecy and praised God, speaking about the baby as the hope of Israel's redemption.

The Bible's words and tone discussing the aging, infirm, orphan, or poor always honors and uplifts them. God identifies with them, calling himself their Father. The Bible never denigrates the weak, frail, or aged. It does confront the corrupt nature within all ages and walks of life—sin is sin, after all—but God never obviates his mercy, love, and justice while doing so. In the biblical worldview, one might argue that at the core, all people are unable to make themselves free of immoral or unjust thoughts and actions (past, present, or future), therefore defining abject spiritual poverty. Thankfully, God proves in word and action his great love for the aged, infirm, orphan, and poor.

God's Provision for the Poor, Aged, and Frail

> Even to your old age and gray hairs
> I am he, I am he who will sustain you.
> I have made you and I will carry you;
> I will sustain you and I will rescue you.
> (Isa. 46:4)

How do the Old and New Testaments refer to the aged? Beyond selecting respectful language when referring to the poor, aged, and frail, God demonstrates his profound concern for them in the way he established and organized the people of Israel. Genesis 2:24 says, "A man will leave his father and mother and be united to his wife, and they will become one flesh." While many have written of this mysterious union, the Hebrew words mean "to cling" or "adhere." From the context of this and other passages, it means that the two are knit together in a family unit. Ideally, they support and cherish each other for life, each giving their all for the other. In this plan, few people will go through life alone.

This presence of two knitted together is clearly by design. It also places the new couple in the context of a greater family that is jointly committed (again, ideally) to helping the members succeed in life. People were designed to be part of mutually beneficial, relational groupings of spouses, families, and communities. And as individuals within the family experience limitations that come from disease or disability as they age, each person retains vital relationships, support, and purpose within the family group.

While corruption is present both within us and any collection of people, the brilliant design of the greater family unit is remarkable. Implicit within the family design is concern and support for the aging and troubled as well as a role and purpose for each person as he or she ages. When families do well, the societies and cultures encourage them to thrive, even when individuals within the families experience frailty, illness, or weakness.

Once the design of family was in place, God created structures regarding how inheritance was to be passed from one generation to another. The Levitical law is unusual in that while addressing how the assets were passed along (as American law does), it also assigns responsibility for who is to ensure the care of the widow, children, or others. In the law, the firstborn son had the responsibility of caring for and protecting the elders, particularly a widow. It could even be extended to a widower unable to make his own way. To help with this and other responsibilities, the law entitled the firstborn to a double portion of any inheritance. In the case that a family had only daughters, the girls received the inheritance so they would have assets and potential income, again to ensure the responsibilities of the entire family were financially supported. The significance of this is that in the law, God made it clear that assets were a tool for the family to benefit one another; people, rather than the assets, were the focus of the inheritance.

God named the patriarch Jacob's sons as Israel's twelve tribes. (This is an oversimplification but it suffices for this discussion.) Each of Jacob's sons had progeny, who later had children, who had children of their own, and so on. Over generations, the tribes grew large and subdivided into smaller groups (clans). So the nation of Israel had twelve tribes, each with several clans to which families identified. Each Jewish family traced its lineage through its clan and tribe to one of the twelve sons of Jacob. Family responsibilities under the Mosaic law were based on the structure of the tribes, clans, and families. Based on that law, the family relation closest to the aged person essentially had the greatest responsibility to look out for their welfare. In that patriarchal society, the law had nuances as to who was the responsible person and how that would at times relate to property ownership. Because they were relatives at some level, tribes, clans, and families were bound to protect and redeem (care for—see also the story of Ruth) one another as needed. Families would know of and be more easily motivated to help those who became infirm or frail (after all, they are family).

While we may perceive this as an anachronism, at that time it meant that every family had an identity and responsibility (purpose) to support their family members, their clan, and their tribe. This structure helped the Jewish nation create and maintain positive social order. For example, an individual in this arrangement would be discouraged from behaving badly (or not caring for an older person) because it reflected poorly on the family, clan, and tribe. Trade and business safely carried on because people could easily learn one another's family and lineage and know who they were working with and their reputation. People knowing one another's business is seen as a privacy issue in our culture; whereas, in a close culture in which relationships prevail, it provides security for the generations.

From our vista of twenty-first-century life, the structure of Israel's law appears to some as a paternalistic anachronism designed to sustain a male-dominated society. The law did presume some separation of roles for men and women but did not subjugate one's value beneath the other. The law called attention to the infirm, aged, and weak to ensure they had protection and dignity. Psalm 19 was written by David, a male king. He called the law perfect, trustworthy, and right, providing refreshment, wisdom, and joy. Beyond some people's judgment on David's ancient poem and the law, look at the greater context of the Bible. Adam and Eve were unique in creation. They were of the same flesh. Equal in relationship, love, dignity, and grace. The law, which came later, clarified roles, never saying that either man or woman was of lessor stature or dignity. In agrarian life, men and women both had life-sustaining and complementary functions. The reality then, as now, people's biases, egos, and need for control and self-preservation created the concepts of lessor and greater worth.

In its perfect form, the Old Testament law protected and dignified those people our culture considers as less important—the aging and others. Jesus came to both fulfill and end the law, but in so doing, he said that the second greatest commandment was to love our neighbors. He did not specify the gender, age, wealth, or social status of that neighbor. Many of the first people attesting about Jesus were women, whose position in society was such that they could not testify as reliable witnesses in court. While the Old Testament law no longer applies, the overarching context of the Bible recognizes the dignity of all people from the garden to God's wedding feast at the end of time. To our shame then, we are the ones who have taken it upon ourselves to treat the aging and others without the dignity God has given them.

Israel's Land Ownership and Its Relations to the Aging

> Blessed are those who have regard for the weak;
> the LORD delivers them in times of trouble.
> The LORD protects and preserves them—
> They are counted among the blessed in the
>   land—
> He does not give them over to the desires of their
>   foes. (Ps. 41:1–2)

In Genesis 12, the Lord called Abram to leave his father's household (family) and go to the land God would show him (Gen. 12:1). When Abram arrived in Canaan, though the Canaanites were in the land at the time, God said, "To your offspring I will give this land" (v. 7). And in Genesis 13:14–15, God again says, "Lift up your eyes from where you are and look north and south, east and west. All the land you see I will give to you and your offspring." When God promised Abram a son, he added, "I am the LORD who brought you out of Ur of the Chaldeans to give you this land to take possession of it" (15:7). Yet again, in Genesis 15:18, the Lord made a covenant with Abram and included, "To your descendants I give this land, from the river of Egypt to the great river, the Euphrates." Finally, in Genesis 17:8, while establishing an everlasting covenant and changing Abram's name to Abraham, God said, yet again, "The whole land of Canaan, where you are now an alien, I will give as an everlasting possession to you and your descendants after you; and I will be their God." God confirmed the oath repeatedly made to Abraham to his son Isaac, "To your descendants I will give all these lands" (26:3). And to Isaac's son Jacob, God said, "I am the LORD, the God of your father Abraham and the God of Isaac. I will give you and your descendants the land on which you are lying" (28:13).

In Genesis 35:9, God changed Jacob's name to Israel, and in verse 12, he said, "The land I gave to Abraham and Isaac I also give to you, and I will give this land to your descendants after you." When Jacob's son Joseph was 110 years old and living with the family in Egypt, where he had cared for them during the great famine, he "said to his brothers, 'I am about to die. But God will surely come to your aid and take you up out of this land to the land he promised on oath to Abraham, Isaac, and Jacob…and then you must carry my bones up from this place'" (50:24). These passages make clear why the Israelites called the place of Canaan "the promised land."

In the 1960s, the movie *Exodus* was made, which depicted the 1948 (most recent) return of the Jews to Palestine. The film's theme song opened with the line, "This land is mine; God gave this land to me." These words refer to God's repeated promise to Israel for the land they occupied for centuries. While many wars and battles have been fought from the time Israel first crossed the Jordan River until now, God's promise and the historical record make it clear why the people of Israel claim the land is theirs. The book of Joshua describes how the land was originally divided in an orderly fashion, tribe by tribe, clan by clan, and family by family. So each person received an allotment of property through the family distribution, which equated to a future and a hope.

Joshua distributed the land to the tribes, clans, and families by lot (described in Joshua 13–21). There is implicit wisdom in dividing the land that way. If the lots were cast fairly, no one could blame the leaders for what property fell to them. As the people of Israel bought and sold land and passed it from each generation to the next, that practice seems consistent with our contemporary practice of land and property transfer. What is different is that in Leviticus 25, God commanded that the entire land was to have a Sabbath rest every seventh year. In that seventh year, according to Deuteronomy 15:1–11, all debts between people were to be canceled. Lenders were expected to be generous to the poor and not be "tightfisted" toward them, particularly as people needing help neared the seventh year Sabbath

(Deut. 15:9–10). Following seven seventh-year Sabbaths (on the fiftieth year), the Year of Jubilee was to be declared (Lev. 25:10–12). Jubilee was to be a holy year, dedicated to the Lord, and crops were not to be planted, all people were to return to their family land, and all property reverted to its original family allotment. Anyone who bought or sold the property between Jubilees was instructed to value the property based on the number of years crops would be harvested before the next Jubilee year (v. 15). Scripture explains the reason for valuing property from Jubilee to Jubilee and its return to the original family groups: "The land must not be sold permanently, because the land is mine and you are but aliens and my tenants. Throughout the country that you hold as a possession, you must provide for the redemption of the land" (vv. 23–24).

Deuteronomy 15 explains the relevance of the land distribution and how it was to remain in each family. "There should be no poor among you, for in the land the LORD your God is giving you to possess as your inheritance, he will richly bless you, if only you obey the LORD your God and are careful to follow all these commands" (v. 4). In verse 11, he says, "There will always be poor people in the land. Therefore, I command you to be openhanded toward your brothers and toward the poor and needy in your land."

By codifying a way for families to lend and borrow money, buy and sell property, and then ensuring the debts will be canceled and property returned generously, God created provision for cash flow to the poor and needy. This encouraged all families to minimize debt and maximize creating value in caring for their property. With property reverting to the original family allotments, families had the opportunity to start over if stricken by difficulty or poverty, and the Year of Jubilee allowed them to start over with debt-free property.

Finally, by allowing both men and women to receive the inheritance of property rights, both genders would have assets available to them if widowed or handicapped in some way. Through this system, God gave his people the means to address and resolve poverty without creating governmental obligation or societal burden while extending the implicit value of the aging in society. In this, he tacitly protects the dignity of each person and refuses to leave them in dire circumstances (unless they refuse to labor for their own benefit). God recognized that the structures he set in place should eliminate or at least diminish poverty in Israel (Deut. 15:4). Yet in verse 11, he acknowledged that there would always be poor because unfortunate situations would occur (effects of corruption). He knew that people would not always fully follow the law's plan and intent to support family members, write off debt, or return property as God directed. Jesus even underscored this to his disciples: "The poor you will always have with you, but you will not always have me" (Matt. 26:11).

God's retention of the ownership of the Promised Land (calling the people of Israel "tenants") indicates His concern for the poor, aged, and frail. How so? First, a landowner (i.e., God) decides how he wants to use his property and is free to select whom he wants to lease his land to. The owner sets the terms under which the land is leased and, subject to the agreement, allows the tenant use of the land. The owner incorporates all the things important to him in the covenants of the agreement, and in accepting it, the owner and tenants each promise to uphold the dictates. The agreement between God and Israel (the covenant and law) was that they could remain on the land so long as they loved and obeyed God. It also covered many different elements, including caring generously for the poor and aging, as well as outlining various festivals and events, such as the Sabbath and Jubilee years. (Some scholars suggest that the years of Israel's enslavement in the captivities equate to the years of Sabbath and Jubilee the nation had failed to observe.) The social structures, laws, and even courts were all part of the plan God laid out for Israel, and it was such to minimize and address the likelihood of poverty and mistreatment of anyone.

Second, God's ownership of the land and valuation of it between harvest years indicated his interest that the land should be fruitful and create a return. God wanted and promised abundant returns to the people as they were faithful and worked the land diligently (Leviticus 25:24: redeeming the land). The people were to work hard to make the land produce. They were to return 10 percent of the bounty as a gift to God (think paying rent to the owner of the land)

and then share portions with the poor. Great harvests (and eventual wealth) would first benefit members of the families, clans, and tribes themselves, and the poor, aged, and frail they supported—meaning that people would not go hungry. God secured the nation's poor and frail with expected generosity and abundant harvests. While it may be easy to let some stranger living in a far-off place go without food, it would be difficult to see an elderly cousin's widow starve when there was plenty to eat, especially when she lived nearby and helped with childcare and other family needs. In one sense you might say that Israel paid a tenth to the owner (God) then used some of the 90 percent they kept to support those near them who were in need.

The instructions God gave Israel were to apply equally to the poor and the alien living among them. So the land was to be worked to create a return. For their part, Israel honored God through caring for people. The outcome of this plan created more recognition and thanksgiving to God from both those benefiting and those creating blessings from his wise plan. In this way, God receives multiple returns on every harvest, and all people were blessed.

Since God owned the property (and it produced abundantly), he could direct the distribution of its crops. As tenants, the Israelites were entitled to the major share of the harvest. In God's economy, he requested only a tenth to be returned to him and asked them to generously share some of their remaining 90 percent with the poor. The tenth returned to God was for the Levitical priesthood and their families, who ministered to the communities as well as serving the poor and infirm. In the sense of a property lease, the redemption price of a tenth plus generosity to the poor does not seem a burden to a sharecropper. Again, this evidences God's compassion for the poor.

How does this discussion of Jewish life and property rights relate to aging? Through his social structures, laws, and blessings, God demonstrates deep care and compassion for the poor. James the brother of Jesus summarizes the law and prophets: "Religion that God our Father accepts as pure and faultless is this: to look after orphans and widows in their distress and to keep oneself from being polluted by the world" (James 1:27). In Israel's culture, the poor were the frail, handicapped, weak, outcast, or alien. Just as in our time, a disproportionate number of their poor were the aged. Injuries and physical limitations hampered people's ability to work, particularly as disabilities increased with age in the physically demanding agrarian society. Sometimes poor business decisions or family dynamics created rifts and isolated individuals (as they do now), and at times, older people would be left alone without property or support.

In times of war, many sons and husbands were lost in battle or limited by injuries, thereby leaving families without laborers. If a man and woman were unable to have children, she lost his income when he died and had to rely on relatives and property value to survive. As is true today, many things can impoverish a person, but the risk increases with age and is compounded by aging's associated health issues and social isolation. Older people's harsh reality is that they may have less physical (and at times cognitive) ability and time to recover from the circumstances causing their poverty.

God set structures in place to protect the widow, the fatherless, and the alien and even directed the courts to equitably resolve legal disputes. The Scriptures called for the courts to treat the poor fairly—not that they were to be given an unfair advantage, but that they were to be heard and all people would receive equal treatment under the law. God wants the frail and poor protected. A prophet reminded Israel of that requirement: "This is what the LORD says: 'Do what is just and right. Rescue from the hands of his oppressor the one who has been robbed. Do no wrong or violence to the alien, the fatherless or the widow, and do not shed innocent blood in this place'" (Jer. 22:3).

Scripture's Language Regarding the Aging

In Deuteronomy, Moses spoke of consequences for Israel if the people did not obey the Lord and observe his commands, such as hunger, thirst, nakedness, poverty, and subservience to another nation, among other things. In the curse, Moses described the character of the enemy Israel would meet: "The LORD will bring a nation against you from far away, like an eagle swooping down, a nation whose language you will not understand, a fierce-looking nation without respect for the old or pity for the young" (Deut. 28:49–50).

The next passages speak of the terrible future the conquering nation would bring against Israel. Note that in the first description of that nation, it speaks not so much of violence as not respecting the old or having compassion on the young. Moses makes it clear that a nation that does not value the aging and young opposes God's plan. Those character traits may be indicators of the evil within those nations.

Notably, the language throughout Scripture describing the treatment of or addressing older people is highly respectful. Words implying that one is losing their faculties, powers, or usefulness due to age are not used in either the Old Testament or the New to describe or address an aging or infirm person. Those negative descriptors are in the Scriptures but are limited to describing something wearing out and are not used to demean an individual. In Matthew 9:16, one does not patch an "old garment" (worn-out garment) with a new patch, or in Ephesians 4:22 where Paul writes, "With regard to your former way of life, put off your old self" (worn-out self or old Adam). Other translations of this and similar passages sometimes use the term translated into English as "old man," but the word describes a worn-out or useless shell rather than denigrating an aging person.

It is startling to realize that the Scriptures do not distinguish between the terms "older person" and "elder." This significantly demonstrates the respect with which the aged were held and carried no negative connotation. The Hebrew word for an older person is *zaqen* and means "elder" or sometimes "senator." Either English term engenders respect and is notably used in Leviticus 19:32, where the people are commanded to stand in the presence of an elder.

The Greek word describing or addressing an older person is *presbuteros*. The word, in its several derivations, occurs over seventy times in the New Testament. It is generally translated as "elder," "ambassador," "of great age," or "senator" (particularly referring to a member of the Jewish ruling council, the Sanhedrin). To many people of our day, the words *old man* or *old lady* conjure multiple images—many of which are negative—but the Scriptures do not portray any negative images regarding aging people. Instead, the language referring to the aged is highly respectful and broadminded.

Think for a moment about the opening illustration of this chapter. What words come to mind as you picture the older woman wearing the long black coat who fell asleep in the crosswalk? What comes to mind after she swings her shopping bag? Do any of the terms you think of or use relate to the word *elder* or *senator*? Our use of language can subtly denigrate people we believe (consciously or subconsciously) are somehow less than us. Consider the forty or more people God used to write the Scriptures. They lived on three different continents in multiple and distinct cultures, wrote in three different languages over fifteen hundred years or so. Yet the congruence of language and respect in the words chosen to depict the poor and the aging is amazingly consistent. Clearly, God wants all people respected but especially elders. Think, too, of the writers of the Scriptures. How many of them had the honor of writing the Scripture through the inspiration of the Holy Spirit only after they were already greatly aged?

Application

God created social and legal structures to ensure that people would care for one another, especially those who were family, alone and without resources to live. Our modern cultural structures differ from the ones prescribed in Jewish law. Reflecting on the Old Testament model underscores a shift in how today's families care for their elders. There is an expectation that protecting the aging is a social responsibility, largely referring to the government and, in part, business or unions. If government regulations assured perfection, then the most highly regulated industry in the country—nursing homes—would be heaven on earth.

The intent of social programs such as Social Security, Medicare, and Medicaid or various pensions is to meet clear needs in our changing culture. Yet government and other institutions' limitations have led our latest generations to take individual responsibility for their own investments. This outlines an ironic duality in our culture: the need for government or others to provide security and assurance contrasted with the distrust that those same institutions have every individual's best interest. For example, Americans demand lower taxes (or to shift the tax burden to others), yet entitlement programs such as Medicare, Medicaid, and Social Security are by far the largest single items in state and federal budgets and are political death to touch. The real costs and demands for elder care and services exceed many families' ability to afford or provide.

Given the complexity of caring for others, it makes sense that God's social structure started with the law's protection of the aging, poor, and infirm. It is better to start with a plan for the elderly and poor rather than addressing that need as an afterthought. Truly, some people's needs went unmet in Israel under the law. The reality is that any system involving humans will be subject to the great corruption in all of us. How do we apply truth in all this? We can start by mirroring God's affection for the aging and poor and ensuring the dignity and honor God bestowed on them. The next time you address an older person, think of referring to them with the words *elder*, *ambassador*, or *senator*. Imagine the impact of expressing that kind of respect could have on the relationship.

Our modern social structure is different from that found in ancient Israel. We have options and ways to serve and care for elders that were unimaginable only a century or two ago. Today's culture is rapidly changing and separating from the biblical roots of those who framed our government. In that change, we face uncharted directions. The Israelites had to feel a similar confusion and concern for the future after leaving behind Egypt's political and social structures. Since we are in a similar situation, we may not be able to change the government or our culture. However, we can do exactly what God taught Israel—to lean on and into him. How do we do that? By trusting him and replicating how God approached the older people in Israel, as reflected in the Bible and the law: with dignity, caring, and by ensuring they had a place and role in each family.

Takeaway Thoughts

Many think that people who lived in earlier centuries had much shorter lives. The truth is, once a person survived childhood and adolescence, their lifespans are more similar to, rather than different from, our modern-day lifespan.

God's law uniquely created a social system for protecting the elderly, young, and infirm. It even returned sold land to the original owners so that poverty might not last for more than one or two generations, if that long. In the days before Christ, holding land, to a large extent, meant life. It was a place for crops, livestock, gardens, and orchards. The law ensured that the land remained in families as it was provided to them. If we are to follow God's lead in loving others and caring for those in need by personal responsibility and structure of our laws, then we are compelled to extend his care and compassion today through both our personal actions and our social systems. One might argue that since all people are created in God's image, respectful treatment of the aged and downtrodden is a logical and expected outcome.

Time and again Scripture speaks of the necessity of protecting old, weak, poor, and infirm people. God's nature is compassionate, and his laws lifted the status of those having little voice. The choice of language regarding the elderly and poor is consistently respectful and honorable.

Questions for Consideration

Immediately after God reminds the people of Israel that the land is his and they are his tenants (Lev. 25:24), he commands them to redeem the land. What does that mean? How did that apply to elders in Israel at the time? How did it apply if an elder was physically unable to work the land?

1. How do our current laws and practices compare with the plan that God laid out for Israel to care for her people?

2. How might the concept of "redeeming the land" apply to our culture? How does it relate to your provision of a place and valuable purpose to the elders in your life?

3. What responsibility has God placed on you for providing for the poor and aged? How might you accomplish that task?

4. What steps can you take to mirror God's respect for the elders in your circle of influence more closely? How do you think those steps would affect the relationship you have with them?

3

Provision for Aging: Gifts

On October 21, 1984, as the nation watched the second presidential debate of the campaign, Henry Trewhitt of the *Baltimore Sun* referred to President Reagan as the oldest sitting president in US history who was tired after the previous presidential debate with Walter Mondale. Trewhitt wondered if Reagan could successfully continue to carry the burden of the high office. Reagan responded in the affirmative and added, "I want you to know that, also, I will not make age an issue of this campaign. I am not going to exploit, for political purposes, my opponent's youth and inexperience."

The focus of this book is moving toward working with or being an elder, and the realities of aging. As discussed earlier, our culture has a fear of aging and sees it as an enemy to be resisted. Or worse, people are to simply be marginalized or even become invisible when reaching a certain age—perhaps Ronald Reagan's age in 1984.

Remember, we were designed to age. Implicit in that creative design are certain gifts and graces that occur only with time. This chapter explores some of the more common strengths and gifts that come through aging. An important key to relating to or becoming an elder, then, is to discover and leverage these strengths and gifts. As Paul described in Romans 12:4–8 and 1 Corinthians 12:4–11, not everyone receives or displays every gift of aging equally or at all, and spiritual gifts from the Holy Spirit are reserved for believers in Jesus. However, in God's creative abundance, we are each designed to be unique, and the mixture of common or spiritual gifts we express as we age underscores our increasing individuality. Rather than discussing the specific gifts of the Spirit, we will look purposefully at the "common" gifts shared by grace to all humanity.

Special giftings that come from the process of living many years—aging—are not the same for all. The expression of any gift we have is developed, at least in part, by focus and improvement of the skill or gift. A basketball player might be "gifted," but talent is developed by practice and training. One could argue that untrained raw talent may not be of value. As we age, we express our gifts in part through experience, but they reach their zenith through individual focus and intentionality. These gifts may best grow through the power of the Holy Spirit as we increase in our knowledge of and love for Jesus.

Aging as Time with God

As a young man in a Bible study on Colossians, I was astounded by the descriptions of Jesus as the firstborn over all of creation. Even more, I began to see his authority over all of creation and how God's fullness was in him. I remarked to an older man who was teaching an adult Sunday school class that the language describing Jesus is amazing. The older man, whose name was Paul (not the one from Scripture—how old do you think I am!) began reciting the section of Scripture I had mentioned. Then he shared deeper truths and observations about that section of Scripture. He was animated by the subject, and it was soon clear to me that his excitement was not from what he could share or that I was looking into that passage; rather, his face brightened because he could speak the truth of how Jesus loved him and loved me. He was excited to talk about a person he knew and loved deeply. On that day I realized I wanted to be like him—maybe not as a biblical scholar but as a man who knows Jesus.

We may perceive a long life as a blessing, as it was for Abraham, Isaac, Jacob, and David—that dying at a good old age is a blessing. But the number of years is not the only blessing; a greater gift is available to us. God wants us to spend time with him in reading, praying, meditating, and participating in other spiritual disciplines. The gift is the outcome of those disciplines. It is not that we are more dearly loved, for we are already loved beyond measure. We eventually become perfect but only in death when we meet him face-to-face (1 John 3:2). We do become more like Jesus, though, as we continue in these practices.

Moses would go up the mountain or enter the tabernacle to meet with God. When he came back from those times, the Israelites could not look at him because his face shone so brightly. They made him wear a veil until the shine wore off. The precious gift God gives his aging people is more time with him to grow in their knowledge of and love for him. This comes through not only the work of the Holy Spirit but also years of abiding with him in his Word. While we do not become perfect, we do begin to reflect his glory in the way we live and through our perspectives and attitudes. Though only as a shadow of him, we begin to share in his character. What an incredible gift!

Aging Typologies as a Gift

You surely have heard the proverb you are only as old as you feel. Surprisingly, the statement implies truth and a common gift.

Gerontologists define age in several ways. Although there are other types of "aging," we will limit our discussion to chronological and physiological aging. The first is chronological age (sometimes called intrinsic aging): how many years a person has lived.

Chronological aging measures the number of days we live. It also describes that at certain times of life, each of us generally experiences similar factors occurring in our bodies and culture. Those things might include common social experiences such as attending school, participating in sports or music, receiving religious education, earning diplomas, getting married, raising children, or retiring. Chronological aging also encompasses a predisposition for genetically driven events (such as puberty and menopause) or disease propensities related, at least in part, to aging, such as certain cancers or heart disease.

The second type of aging is physiological aging, at times called extrinsic or environmental aging. This is to say that some people age physically faster than others, and the body can be older or younger than the average person of the same chronological age. Smoking cigarettes, not exercising, and overconsumption of alcohol generally causes the body to fail faster than the body of those who regularly engage in healthier behavior. Physiological aging suggests that our genes react to certain health and environmental factors we put our bodies through. Again, smoking and lack of exercise somehow force our genes to respond in certain ways while eating healthy foods, regular exercise, and engaging in meaningful socialization encourage our genes to act in different ways. Simply put, we are stewards of our bodies, and we generally reap the rewards or consequences of how we treat our bodies.

Because of the corruption of our original design, this stewardship is not entirely formulaic, but it is a general pattern for life. This physical stewardship may increase the number of days we experience but, just as important may also improve the quality of our last days. In the book *Live Long, Die Short*, Dr. Landry cites research showing that quality of late life is somewhat a product of genetics, while the stewardship of our physical selves is up to us.[1] The better we steward our physical, mental, social, and spiritual selves, the more likely we will remain vibrant and engaged much closer to when we die.

It is noteworthy that this "stewardship" is remarkably like the activities called out earlier in this book describing the culture and way of life God designed for the Jewish community and family (keeping familial and cultural roles for the aging, ensuring the firstborn son's responsibility for caring for the parents, and creating food and physical security for the aged and infirm through leaving of portions of the harvest, etc.). This is illustrative of how our Creator understands how he designed us and how we best function. These stewardship activities are encouraged even more in the economy of God's grace because they are based in love. God's unfathomable love and acceptance of us increase the physiological and psychological impact of our stewardship as we grow in the knowledge and application of the gospel's redemption. Who among us cannot be happy, fulfilled, and giving knowing we are forgiven, immeasurably loved, desperately wanted, and completely accepted? Consider the effect of that reality on the elder who daily lived out that truth for decades. It is a gift far more certain than a simple positive outlook might attain.

People often say that they feel many years younger than their chronological ages. Though in their minds they feel forty or fifty years old, this thinking contributes to their seventy-year-old (or older) bodies suffering injuries. Climb a ladder? No problem…until the aging body is unable to keep its balance. Exercise is a good idea, but not so much after being away from the gym for twenty years and the meniscus or rotator cuff tears from poor equipment use, not starting gradually, or failure to stretch adequately. A dad with heart problems and a pack-a-day smoking habit decided to start jogging with his son to build "his wind back." It is easy to guess what happened in that case. In aging, people often believe they are stronger and less vulnerable than they are—perhaps because emotions and self-perception do not age in the way the physical body does.

This sense of not aging can hold true even for people with severe memory loss and who often believe they are decades younger than their chronologies. Some elders suffering from severe memory loss do not recognize the older person they see in a mirror because they believe themselves to be decades younger. Have you noticed that, unless you are in pain or have a major health issue, you do not "feel" as old as your chronological age? This is not to suggest that you have early memory loss, but it does point to a quiet truth at work within us: this sense of being younger than our physical ages suggests that our thoughts and emotions do not age as rapidly as our physical bodies. Since most people experience this, it could be a created design element we share. While it can lead us into difficulty (e.g., playing basketball with teenagers might not be a good idea for a fifty-year-old), it can provide pathways for us to remain engaged across the generations.

The dichotomy between how old our bodies are and how we feel has unexpected benefits. First, it supports the processes that make each of us more "ourselves" as we age. We are each unique in personality and genetic mix at birth—those things that define us. Though our general traits remain pretty much the same throughout life, they are moderated by life experiences, successes, and failures alike. Thus, to my wife's chagrin, I will likely always enjoy puns and see them everywhere. On the other hand, my wife's gift of ignoring my extreme wit will continue to build her character. This demonstrates how my wife and I are becoming more distinct and like "ourselves" through life. One result of aging is that we become more unique as we age; thus, we have more individual perspectives that can apply to growing in wisdom and insight.

Second, as we become more unique, we also grow in our sense of independence. Since we generally feel younger than our age, and we see ourselves as vibrant individuals, we fiercely defend our independence and the purposes we select for ourselves. This self-perception may explain why some people remain in jobs longer than they may be effective, fulminating against anyone suggesting they can no longer do the work. It is the same mindset of an older person whose strength or balance diminishes, risking a dangerous fall. Denial of the current reality is common (since we all do it to some degree), and we vigorously defend our independence. This self-independence can be disastrous in the presence of a lone person's short-term memory deficit. Yet it is a powerful motivator for many elders that younger caregivers can leverage to help guide elders toward healthy lifestyles. It is powerful when an elder discovers that using a device or tool, such as a cane or night lighting, can help him or her retain independence.

Third, our emotions appear to remain undiminished through life. Elders experience the full range of emotions they had in their youth. They are tempered, however, by experience and what they consider socially appropriate. Elda was a proud and gracious woman who did not cry at her husband's funeral. She told me that we are not to show sadness in church. Elda did weep privately with her daughters and as she grieved in her room. "Age does not diminish the extreme disappointment of having a scoop of ice cream fall from the cone," says Jim Fiebig. This quote (from Goodreads) puts it succinctly. People in their eighties still feel a full range of emotion; they may become giddy in love like a twenty-year-old or incensed at a price increase. The depth of grief and loss of a spouse or a child does not diminish with age. Older couples in their courtship and romance are fun to be with because they are so alive and in love. The happiness they experience in a long-awaited wedding or newborn grandchild is just as joyful as it would have been twenty or forty years earlier. The difference in how emotions may be expressed is tempered by the experiences and social beliefs of an older person. The expression of emotions may be different between generations, cultures, experiences, or time periods. As we age, our depth of feeling, whether ecstatic, happy, sad, or depressed, remains the same regardless of its expression.

Elders who recognize emotions they and others experience often exhibit the gift of readily listening to and understanding others' difficulties in life. It may contribute to why grandchildren sometimes relate deeply with grandparents because they are met with understanding by people who have the gift of time to listen.

Lifestyle Adaptation as a Gift

Another gift of aging is that our bodies defer to our lifestyles. Conceptually, our bodies tend to adapt to the life we live. When I was in my twenties, I watched a crew of bricklayers build a concrete wall brick by brick. The bricklayers were from a small but highly recommended family company. The owner was in his sixties and spent his days in the trenches, laying heavy concrete blocks with his workers. I was amazed that he had the strength and stamina to heft block all day long. He had started doing brickwork in high school and never stopped for over forty years. He was slender, wiry, and filled with vitality. While he certainly had a good genetic mix for that work, the work itself affected his life. It gave him a daily workout, and to do the work he loved, he had to take care of himself. His love for his work both encouraged and aided him to be a good steward of his physical body.

People living on the east side of Cleveland, Ohio, know about lake-effect snow. When the conditions are right, the snow is distributed in massive, heavy wet cold drifts on top of thick layers of slush. It weighs too much for a small snowblower, so clearing a driveway becomes a daunting project requiring heavy-duty shovels and a lot of sweat. But cold air constricts our blood vessels, so the collision of seasonal hard manual labor, the constriction of blood vessels, and the added stress of hard work result in repetitive motion injuries and many heart attacks. If people were to work like this every few days, thus training their bodies, they could adapt and help them through it because shoveling and throwing wet snow is a type of intense weight training. But for many people, manual labor, like shoveling snow, is not a regular part of their lifestyles. In short, their bodies have not adapted to the physical effort, and to take it on suddenly without preparation causes their bodies to fail. Peoples' bodies adapt to a less rigorous lifestyle when they do not regularly perform the level of exertion readying them to shovel heavy, wet snow. Our bodies adjust to how we live.

A large and growing body of research is studying the long-term impact of how we treat our bodies over our lifetimes. Researchers note that aging professors often can remain current and relevant in their selected fields well into their seventies, eighties, and some even beyond. People with healthy diets tend to maintain physical health for longer periods than those who abuse alcohol or drugs for years. It makes sense that there is a benefit of being good stewards of our bodies. The point here is not to recount the material readily available elsewhere but to underscore that our bodies defer to our lifestyles. That means they gradually change to support the lives we live.

So if we change our lifestyles, our bodies respond. For example, if a person gives up cigarettes after years of smoking, their bodies will recover some of what was lost. Usually, pundits argue that healthy living adds years to life. Scripture teaches us that God has already numbered our days (Job 14:5; Ps. 37:18, 139:15–18). If our days are numbered, then what is the value of being good stewards of our bodies? The simple answer is that the better we treat our bodies, the stronger they will be, allowing us to live well until the day we die. It is an issue of enhancing the quality of life for every day we live. Good stewardship helps us to be vibrant and thrive in each of our days. As good physical stewards, we will be most able to exercise choice and pursue our desires and purposes for as long as possible.

Experience and Wisdom as a Gift

With age comes the gift of experience. That gift is generally expressed in two main ways with a third expression being "optional."

The first expression of experience is the imprinting of memories of our experiences. This history is as unique as each of us, all colored with the perspective of our situations. Elders can tell you where they were and what their experience was in both personal as well as public events such as when President Kennedy was assassinated, or while viewing the grainy images of the first moon walk, or the aircraft flying into the Twin Towers in New York City. The history each of us carries makes great conversation and discovery as we learn one another's places in history. Hearing about an elder's personal experience during times of historical significance brings those events alive in ways that highlight both the person and the larger events.

How should wisdom be defined? In ancient Hebrew, the word we translate as "wisdom" more deeply means "skill in living." The first painting a future Master artist creates is not a masterpiece. Masterpieces are created following years of focus, practice, failure, and developing innate skills. Wisdom is the same, in that years of thoughtful practice in life with success and failure creates skill in living. Of course, some people seem to be more skilled than others, but even for them, the ultimate skill in living is not proven until they have accumulated years of experience.

Many people who experience memory loss lose their most recent memories first. Long-term memories are usually retained longer. This tendency explains why the history from an elder's early life may remain even while current events are lost. Rekindling events from their early lives is one way to stay in touch with an older person who has memory loss; this can help maintain the relationship as well as create legacy moments for younger generations. Take care, though, to rekindle only those memories that bring desirable experiences and emotions to the surface. (Indiscriminate probing of an individual's past can unexpectedly unearth early childhood traumas and abuse, even though they occurred eighty years earlier, and the emotional response may still arise.)

Second, with experience comes the knowledge of situations and what was successful. Call this skill in living—traits that each of us develops through good and bad experiences over time. It is like the story of a young man taking over a retiring CEO's job. The young man asked the outgoing retiree how to be successful in the role. The older man replied, "Good decisions."

"But how," the young man said, "do I learn to make good decisions?"

The older man stopped at the exit, turned, and peered into the young man's eyes. "Bad decisions."

We grow as we apply what we learn through experiences. Since older people have more years of life, they have this gift of experience. When facing a new concern, they often consider how prior experiences may apply and respond in a manner consistent with the earlier event.

When discussing aging, it is common to hear, "with age comes wisdom." This is the third gift of experience, and it is optional. Saying that every person over seventy-five is wise is like saying that all houses have basements. Not every house is guaranteed to have a basement. Elders all have skill in living to a greater or lesser degree from their experiences and their early influencing adults (parents, teachers, etc.). But just because a person has life experience and knowledge does not mean he will either learn from the experiences or find ways to apply them. Many older people lived through the various economic downturns that guide them toward conservative planning and living. Others who lived through the same economic upsets still experience surprising financial losses when another recession occurs. This is wisdom gleaned from the combination of experiences filtered by circumstances and personality while living in the world.

The highest value of experience is found in another form of wisdom. Scriptures point to wisdom from the fathers (things we learn from teachers, mentors, etc.), from our experiences (as described above), and from our heavenly Father. In his ancient primer on wisdom, Job wrote, "To God belong wisdom and power; counsel and understanding are his" (Job 12:12–13). The point is that in addition to all of his other attributes, God is wise. His wisdom is greater than our application of experience, and it looks different from skill in living. Job says, "The fear of the Lord—that is wisdom, and to shun evil is understanding" (28:28). The apostle Paul wrote the following:

> Where is the wise man? Where is the scholar? Where is the philosopher of this age? Has not God made foolish the wisdom of this world? For since in the wisdom of God the world through its wisdom did not know him, God was pleased through the foolishness of what was preached to save those who believe. (1 Cor. 1:20)

And then again:

> We do, however, speak a message of wisdom among the mature, but not the wisdom of this age or of the rulers of this age, who are coming to nothing. No, we speak of God's secret wisdom, a wisdom that has been hidden and that God destined for our glory before time began. (1 Cor. 2:7)

The wisdom of God comes from the Father through his Holy Spirit. And this gift comes as we know and experience him in life. It comes as a gift through years of intimate times with him, through the struggles and trials of life. Apparently, it has eternal benefit, which is not entirely clear on this side of eternity.

Legacy as a Gift

"[A prophecy and blessing to Jacob]: You, however, will go to your ancestors in peace and be buried at a good old age" (Gen. 15:15).

Experience has a companion gift: legacy. The history of a family is inextricably bound within the elder. Only he or she carries the stories and knowledge of who the family is and how the family came to be. Each of us longs to know that we "fit" within a context and family legacy that provides security and purpose. Family and community fill this need, and elders within our relations can create a sense of family through shared legacy.

An attribute associated with legacy is a concept called "generational complementarity," a term coined by Vickie Rosebrooke, PhD, a friend and colleague. She researched the relationship between elders and young children in a day care in a Northwest Ohio nursing home. She observed and researched the idea that elders and young children have complementary needs and strengths. For example, elders have time, the desire to share experiences, and the need to share themselves with others (an aspect of purpose). Youth have energy, the need to learn to respect, a desire to hear stories, and an ability to look beyond physical limitations. When structured in a healthy environment, the children's needs are met simultaneously with the elders' needs. The needs and strengths of each group complement and meet the needs and strengths of the other.

Generational complementarity can help explain a designed plan for the sharing of experience and legacy while simultaneously granting purpose and joy to both generations. A disproportionate number of people working in elder services today will point to an elder they became close to while growing up—a beneficiary of generational complementarity that is passed on through their work with elders.

Not all elders enjoy being with young children, but many do and find it a great source of encouragement. Even very frail older people can greatly benefit from engaging with a child or teen relationship. The key is to focus on creating relationships. For example, having children go to a nursing home to sing songs or do plays is enjoyable for older people. However nice the entertainment is, relationships have far more life-changing effects than entertainment alone. This fact is easily illustrated. How many people attend school events and concerts of young children when they do not know any of the children? Very few because there is little return for the experience for the children or adults. However, if a parent's child is in a choir, play, or sports event, most parents will attend. Why? In some ways, the experience together builds on and enhances the relationship. The need for multigenerational relationships does not change with age.

The gift of legacy implicitly shares the experiences of an older group of people (but not necessarily wise) with a cohort, who learns through stories and common views. This influence passes on the elders' perceptions of the world to the younger generations and creates dialogue and learning. While frequently maligned as being "old-fashioned" by younger generations, insight created through life produces experience not necessarily conservativism. Often experience has taught elders to be more open to the truth than the younger generations. In John 8, a woman caught in the act of adultery was brought before Jesus. The Pharisees said the law required that she be stoned and, intending it as a trap, asked Jesus what he thought. Jesus taught them a greater truth by saying that the person without sin should throw the first stone. "At this those who heard it began to go away one at a time, the older ones first." Why did the older ones go first? They were not necessarily more sinful but were more honest with themselves and, in that circumstance, more willing to acknowledge the truth about themselves regardless that the challenge came from Jesus.

Elders bring a testimony to the faithfulness and constancy of God as well as the reliability of his promises. History is replete with examples of elders being the first to see and act on truth that younger people were unwilling or unable to accept. In these cases, elders brought important influence to teach younger generations through powerful words and actions.

Our perspective of time changes as we age. Many older people I have known say that time seems to accelerate as we age. They have said, as the psalmist wrote, we begin to see "The length of our days is seventy years—or eighty, if we have the strength; yet their span is but trouble and sorrow, for they quickly pass, and we fly away" (Ps. 90:10). Though time quickly goes, our changing sense of time is a gift to the aging as well. There is wisdom in numbering our days because as we age, we often have less strength and stamina to do things we always have done. This compels us to reset our lifestyles and priorities, creating available time from formerly busy and unconsidered lives. Time, as a gift, helps us to live and love in the present and makes each moment count even when they are ones of trouble or sorrow. This gift of time helps us focus on creating a legacy while freeing us to seek our daily purpose and refreshment in the Lord, who loves us tenderly.

At the end of life, people often discard the unimportant and embrace that which holds the greatest value to them. In nursing homes, elders near death often say that they value family most, followed by those they were able to help, or helped them, through life. I have known many, many people who died during my forty-year career, and none have wanted more money, prestige, or possessions. While some asked for more time, there was a caveat to the request: they wanted more time to be with the people they loved. In these, the most courage I have ever seen is those elders who live with dignity and integrity into the time of their deaths. It seems to be a gift available after living a life of character and faith. People who are the most intimate with the Lord have a peace and sense of joy in that death. That, too, is a gift, lesson, and legacy to grow into while we yet have years before us.

Courage as a Gift

There is courage among the elders who seek the best and growth in others, even when they themselves are in active decline. They recognize the value in people and encourage them to love completely and with abandon. The gift of this courage is a certainty in their purpose to love and provides a sense of purpose, peace, and calm throughout the last years. There is no bluster or bragging in this type of courage; it is an attractive, encompassing trait that draws people to the elder.

A young boy insisted on seeing his "Grand-friend," who was in the hospice area of a nursing home and was actively dying, only hours to live. The family refused to let the boy visit until the elder whispered for him by name. As he had done many times before, the boy quietly climbed onto her bed, gently hugged his friend, and placed his head with one ear against her chest as she held him. After a while, he raised up and said, "She still has a good heart." She died quietly an hour after he left. He will never forget her.

Frankness as a Gift

The final gifts many consider not to be gifts at all. Many elders become less self-conscious about how they speak to others. It is as if they are completely open about what they think—often without any kind of social filter on their choice of language. This is a gift because when working with an elder who is like this, it is easy to know what he thinks or what she feels. I played guitar in a coffee house once, and an older woman walked out, loudly saying, "This guy is awful." I knew then that I needed to work on my skills and broaden my music's appeal.

As refreshing as receiving a true opinion can be, this guileless-ness can be an issue in a couple of ways. First, it can hurt peoples' feelings. The way we deal with that is by being adults and address the issue or concern in a straightforward but respectful way. Elders are adults, fully entitled to their opinions, but as adults they are also responsible for how they treat others. At times, frank comments are made in an overloud fashion simply because the speaker has some hearing loss.

Another issue with the frank comments provides clues to what may be happening deep inside the person's brain. Many factors affect how the brain functions and ages. And many things can cause a person's brain not to work properly, including medications, stress, nutrition, environment, genetics, and organic brain disease—some are treatable, if not reversible. One way the brain can "misfire" is when involved factor(s) affect the frontal lobe of the brain (basically behind the forehead). While there are several functions of the frontal lobe, one is the center that drives impulse control, which is the brain's function that keeps us from speaking or doing inappropriate or risky things and helps us maintain social equilibrium. It is also one of the later things to develop in a child's brain and may explain some of the risky behavior of the mid and late teen years (particularly in males). Impulse control is like a filter that helps us navigate through life safely and within social norms. Impeding the filter of impulse control can result in a loss of social appropriateness and, occasionally, modesty.

As already mentioned, this may be a signal that changes are occurring in the brain that may be reversible with proper diagnosis and treatment. If an elder's personality or impulse filter changes, it is wise to seek a medical evaluation with the greatest potential for improvement or minimization if treated early. For some, frankness is an indicator of changes inside the brain; for others, though, it may be a deliberate decision to just be honest and direct. My mom once said a friend "was tired of people's crap" and was not going to put up with it any longer. Her friend's life experience led her to deliberately change how she dealt with people—a rational life choice.

Other changes in the brain can cause a variety of issues for elders. For example, the same part of the brain that helps us remember hymns also appears to store inappropriate words. A person with significant memory loss may still sing every verse of an old hymn while unable to remember a loved one's name or suddenly come out with swear words she never used as an adult. While I cannot explain how this happens, evidently the grace of God in remembering beautiful music and our corrupt natures battle each other even when our memories fail.

A key point to remember, though, is that when the brain fails, the love of Jesus does not. Though the person we remember may not be apparent to us, God knows, remembers, and values him. In his commitment to Jesus, nothing can separate him from God's love and salvation (Psalm 139, Isaiah 49:15–18, Romans 8:18–39).

Humility as a Gift

A widely perceived reality is that as many people age, their worlds become smaller. Think about it. My wife and I had a 3,600 square foot house, and we realized that having all that space was unnecessary when our children live elsewhere. We found a much more convenient home with a first-floor master bedroom of about 2,500 square feet. I know of a woman who is downsizing from an 8,000 square foot house to 1,200 square feet. Someone moving to assisted living will have about 500 to 800 square feet. A nursing home may relegate them to 100 or 120 square feet. On the face of it, downsizing does not reflect humility. However, what is the nature of downsizing? It is a gradual process of setting priorities on the things we cherish and want to keep near us.

Downsizing can force us to recognize the reality that our identities lie outside what we believe defines us. It is far easier to accept the smaller spaces when the elder considers this option in advance. An unintended move from a 2,500 square foot house to 500 square feet in an assisted living or 150 square feet (or less) in a nursing home is humiliating for people, particularly when their identity is tied in with their homes that they lived in and cherished for many years.

Two things seem to be the most valuable to people as they age: pictures and relationships. The pictures may provide memories of times gone by—what parent in later years does not look wistfully at images of their young children or beloved family and friends, some of whom may have passed away? Or sometimes they miss a favorite pet or place where they had great memories (usually with other people).

This may make you sad (compassion is in us all), but notice the other "thing" that remains is relationships—both former and current. Humility? No, but consider this. When our personal "worlds" shrink, the parts that remain are who we have become and our relationships, regardless if we live in a mansion or a shared bedroom in a nursing home. People around an elder may ask, "Who was he?" or "Who was she?" The influence we have on others is generally absent of many forms of power—sometimes even memory or the ability to speak. So how do we come to see ourselves as we connect with others in an arena where status and strength are curtailed?

Some elders try to force others to do what they want through volume or sheer unpleasantness. Others see themselves as victims and helpless. It can be argued that aging people who thrive, especially in their latest years, are those who express kindness, thoughtfulness, peace, patience, goodness, and self-control in relation with others— ultimately thinking of others as important. This is the art of engaging others and influencing them through the gift of humility.

An eighty-six-year-old woman was dying. She had served for decades as a highly educated and respected RN. The doctors and she knew that her death would be sometime in the following several months. She was able to get around and meet people in her assisted living building while remaining in hospice. She had befriended one of her caregivers who had emigrated to the United States and spoke thickly accented broken English. The caregiver confided to the older woman that she wanted to become a certified nurse's aide so she could better her life. The older woman asked what was keeping her from following her passion. The caregiver replied that she could not read English well enough to take the course and pass the test. The older woman taught the caregiver to read. At the older woman's funeral, the caregiver said that she would never forget the kindness this highly educated woman had shared with her to sit and teach her to read. She said, also, that she learned so much more than just how to read. The older woman had shared her last days with the caregiver with no expectation in return. This is the power of the gift of humility.

Compassion as a Gift

The last gift we will discuss is one I call the gift of the dentist (apologies to my dentist friends). When I was young, visiting the dentist was an experience forced upon me by my parents and accompanied by my trepidation. I almost always had cavities, and the repairs were smelly, loud, and painful affairs. When young, I did not understand my parents' value in the dentist. Although my parents had little money, they made sure that all four of their children visited the dentist regularly. Mom and Dad put up with the squawking and whining as an act of something to benefit us later. They may have felt bad about my tears and pain and listened to all of my excuses and rational arguments for not seeing the dentist. Yet they prevailed, and off I went…because they loved me. That is the point: sometimes compassion does not dress in fancy garb; sometimes it is hidden inside something we deem painful.

Compassion expressed is an action to benefit another person, often at personal cost to the one showing the care. It turns out that making me go to the dentist was a compassionate act of my parent's sacrificial love. Going to the dentist was a blessing, of course, because I expect to keep my teeth well into my elder years, so long as I continue the self-discipline of routinely visiting the dentist. Today dentistry is far more sophisticated and less uncomfortable, though I still get a little nervous going for routine appointments. This "visiting the dentist" gift from my parents blesses me every time I eat (which is frequent), though while growing up, the "visits" made for the most dreaded of days.

In Mark 1:40–41, Jesus is met by a man with leprosy (or a terrible skin disease). The man said, "If you are willing, you can make me clean." Before Jesus reaches out his hand and heals the man, Mark describes Jesus's response in three words: "Filled with compassion." In Greek, the phrase infers that Jesus was deeply moved, moved to the inner depths of himself. Jesus was not flippant or matter-of-fact, and he was not merely empathetic or "professional" (which is how modern health-care workers are trained: empathy, yes; sympathy, no). Jesus was moved with compassion for a man he had never met and who simply asked him for help. The operative gift here for us is compassion.

While some of us express compassion more naturally, compassion does not abound in nature. Compassion is God's specific attribute shared a bit in nature (perhaps in nurturing young or injured animals), but when He designed us in his image (Gen. 1:26–27), he doused us with the ability to see and act compassionately. Time and again God describes the compassion he has for us. Psalm 91:4 says, "He will cover you with his feathers and under his wings you will find shelter." Or look at Isaiah 49:15–16: "Can a mother forget the baby at her breast and have no compassion on the child she has borne? Though she may forget, I will not forget you! See, I have engraved you on the palms of my hands."

God is the author of compassion, and according to what Paul wrote to the Ephesians and elsewhere, God is developing in each of us his character as we walk with him. That means we learn and increase our compassion through knowledge of and experience with God as he guides and molds us through the Holy Spirit.

Compassion is more than a deep feeling. It compels action, as it did of Jesus with the leper in Mark 1. We know Jesus acted on his compassion more often than what Mark recorded in his first chapter. We know this because the Scriptures reveal often that Jesus was "moved." Compassion motivated Jesus to climb onto the cross, and it defines him in his resurrected state today.

Compassion ultimately cost Jesus his life, and perhaps this is the best depiction of complete compassion. Yet compassion is primarily known in the context of those needing or benefiting from it. Compassion grows as we use it with others.

While aging itself can be challenging, we would do well to consider that compassionately aiding the aging and others in their difficulties is a gift and blessing to us as we learn to be more compassionate by exercising compassion. It is blessed to share in God's compassion, and caring for the frail, the helpless, the ill, the poor, and the orphan and widow develops, exercises, and proves the gift of compassion within us. Building that gift and character within us is often difficult and at times costly; in it we share in the sufferings of Jesus. It is only in seeing God's compassion that we become aware of that aspect of his character. Then sharing compassion causes us to become more compassionate people.

As we age, we receive and then uniquely express the gifts of aging. The gifts include believing we are younger than our chronology claims. We gain experience, knowledge, and insight that transcend the decades, culminating in the gift of wisdom for some. We learn to offer the gift of legacy and seek opportunities to pass it on to upcoming generations, learning through the length of life what is important. Courage is often a gift to elders who teach those closest to them to observe and learn how to live with dignity and grace. Some elders receive the gift of frankness—openness of thought and concept plainly stated to cut through the detritus of life. Some of us can grasp humility as a gift to profoundly affect others we relate with. Then, finally, living and working with elders and others in need may, at times, force us to confront our need to grow in the practice of expressing compassion. This gift given to us has great benefit for both those receiving our compassion and us as we grow through expressing it.

These gifts help define who we are becoming and teach us to identify and value what is important and lasting. Ultimately, the gifts help us to grow through life and then express and face our humanity. For believers, these gifts help to define who we are.

Application

The process of aging offers certain gifts to each of us. Using the foundation of purpose and respect discussed in earlier chapters, can you recognize the gifts of elders near you? Can you identify how the gifts of aging are causing you to grow and change? How has the hand of God worked in your life through time?

Have you met an elder who possesses godly wisdom? How did he or she express that gift? How might that gift be developed and encouraged in your growth?

How many people can you name from the Bible whom God specifically used in old age (other than the patriarchs and Moses)? Hint: Anna, Zacharia, and Elizabeth. But who else? Why is it significant that God used them in their old age?

Takeaway Thoughts

God grants certain gifts to us—each in its own time. While some people speak of being endowed with youth and vigor, most people do not recognize that aging itself offers gifts that come only with time lived.

God loves his servants here on earth, and a blessing of long life is the opportunity to spend more time with God: knowing him personally and deeply. Because he is infinite in grace, love, and mystery, we can never know everything about him in our lifetimes. He uses the mystery of himself to draw us closer to him as the years go on.

It is reassuring that as we age, we become "more like ourselves." Our personalities and personhood remain, as do our memories and important aspects of our identification. We feel younger than our chronology, and it is encouraging!

The gifts of wisdom, legacy, courage, frankness, humility, and compassion are honed through the process of aging. These gifts are not given equally to all, and they do not develop without our participation. As we learn of God and exercise these gifts, they grow as God desires.

Questions for Consideration

1. If the word *wisdom* in the Hebrew means "skill in living," how might an elder's skill in living be helpful for you?
2. What is your family's history? Can you relate your ancestors' experiences and wisdom stories? Do you think they demonstrated skill in living through their stories?
3. Have you ever been uncomfortable because of the frankness of an older person? Do you think the elder was correct in his or her comment? How did you handle the experience?
4. Of wisdom, legacy, courage, frankness, humility, and compassion, which gifts are developing in your life?
5. How do you typically think of courage? What does it look like in an older person you know?
6. Do you consider humility to be a gift? Why or why not?
7. Have you reflected on God's compassion to help you grow in your sense of compassion for others? Do you think you have more compassion for others today than you did five or ten years ago because of your relationship with God? Why or why not? What can you do to be more compassionate?
8. Compassion is a character trait specifically used by God to describe himself. As with all gifts of God, some are easier to express and act on than others. Reflect on the difference between feeling compassion and acting on it. How is God challenging you to grow in your exercise of this important trait? What acts of compassion come to mind that you could express toward others?
9. How might you use your knowledge of elders and the gifts of aging to leverage a better relationship with the elders you know?

4

Promoting an Elder's Interests: The Advocate

Speak up for those who cannot speak for themselves,
for the rights of all who are destitute.
Speak up and judge fairly; defend the rights of the poor and needy.
—Proverbs 31:8–9

The Old Testament story of Ruth shows the structure of Jewish law and society in the way a man named Boaz served as an advocate. Boaz was a relative of an older widow, Naomi, and, by default, her daughter-in-law Ruth. Under the law and social structure, relatives had a responsibility to care for one another. The closer the relation, the greater the responsibility.

Because of a famine in Bethlehem, Elimelech had moved his wife, Naomi, and their two sons to Moab, where they lived for several years. The sons took Moabite women for wives. Sadly, Elimelech and his sons died, leaving Naomi and her daughters-in-law widowed.

When Naomi learned that the famine in Israel had ended, she decided it was time to return to her homeland in Bethlehem. Her daughter-in-law Ruth went with her, even though it meant she would face many obstacles. Yet her story is awe-inspiring when you consider that she

- was raised a Moabite, whom Jews disparaged;
- was childless (in that culture, to be childless was to be without a lineage and outside of God's blessing); and

- was widowed, with no one to provide for her.

Yet she threw her lot in with her impoverished mother-in-law. Most important was that Ruth became a Jew by choice when she committed her life to Naomi and Naomi's God.

In Bethlehem, Naomi had rights through the family line to a parcel of land. Recall in the earlier chapter where we discussed that the land was originally given by God, ordained to the tribes, clans, and families, and was to remain in the family's ancestral line in perpetuity. The line would pass from one generation to another through inheritance. Land could be sold but only to relatives, and in the Year of Jubilee, it was to return to the original family.

Boaz, a distant relative of Naomi, saw Ruth, knew who she was, and honored Ruth and Naomi by supplying food, respect, and protection for them. He helped them because he was an honorable man and loved the Lord and his law. When Ruth approached him for marriage—at Naomi's instruction—he seemed surprised, yet pleased, since she had caught his eye.

Before Boaz could marry Ruth, he had to discuss the purchase of Naomi's land with her closest relative, who had first rights. The purchase of the land meant the original lineage went with the property. Thus, Naomi and Ruth would become the new owner's responsibility, including producing an heir to preserve the ancestral line. In other words, the relative who purchased the land would have to marry Ruth, and if she bore children, any heirs from the marriage would have rights to Naomi's property in addition to participating fully in any inheritance the new husband might bring to the marriage.

Naomi's closest relative declined the "offer." That suited Naomi, Ruth, and Boaz, for Boaz wanted to marry Ruth and gladly took the responsibility to provide for and protect Naomi too.

Boaz acted as an advocate for Naomi and Ruth at not only personal expense but also social risk for marrying a childless, Moabite woman who had become a Jew. Since she had been barren in her earlier marriage, there was a risk that they might not be able to produce heirs. This was a far greater risk than is evident in our culture today.

Boaz provides an excellent example of an advocate taking multiple risks and potential future costs to care for others. His reward was becoming the grandfather of King David and a direct ancestor of the ultimate advocate, Jesus.

The Scriptures often speak of the "needy." The younger me thought that "needy" meant not having money. Of course, now I realize my mistake. A better definition is that *needy* means "not having the resources to overcome a situation or being helpless in certain circumstances." Need, in that sense, may be money, food, support, socialization, help with taxes…or any number of things. For example, God knew our *need* before we existed and sent Jesus to address our helplessness.

Advocacy is to plead the cause of another person who is unable to sufficiently plead his or her own cause or protect themselves. As a loving advocate, God is always looking out for our best interests as he writes our lives as subplots within his story.

A crucial part of being an advocate is to take on the perspective of the person being advocated. Advocates should always work to preserve the dignity of the people for whom they advocate and should not presume to know the other's mind. Without first understanding the recipient's perspective, the advocate's approach and solutions may be woefully unsuccessful. The advocate must always think about what the person needing help is experiencing and wants. To the extent that is reasonable, advocates should try to maximize the autonomy and decisions for the people they support. What they want may not be what they actually need, but knowing them, their history, and their mind supplies clues to how advocates should proceed.

The long-term relationship between the advocate and the elder can make the advocate's role difficult, particularly when she has a strong emotional connection with the elder. Even when the advocate and elder agree about difficult decisions those choices can be emotionally laden. The advocate's emotional cost increases commensurately when she does not agree with the elder's choices. I love my mom and did not want to see her prolong her health issues. Yet she was ready to die and wanted no part in curative care (though there was none available). Contacting hospice was her decision, and a wise one. Yet for me, as one of her advocates and a professional in the field, my emotions were conflicted between her choice and my desire to keep mom in my life. Whether the advocate's and elder's decisions agree or not, the role will be emotionally draining at times. Later, however, advocates often find the blessings and satisfaction gained far outweigh the emotional toll.

Advocacy may take many different forms ranging from meeting medical, social, emotional needs or to creating connections, but is always focused on the best interest of the one needing support. Some examples might be, a man with cognitive limits constantly requested to go to his longtime home. His family took him there, but he did not recognize it as his. He may have been expressing is that he was feeling lost, disconnected from what was familiar to him. What did the family do? They took him out for mint chocolate chip ice cream, his favorite. And for that short time, he seemed more relaxed and like himself. Later, they brought his dog to visit with him. He could not remember the dog's name, but on some level, he reconnected with his pet.

Susan, an older woman had transportation issues. Her neighbor planned to drive Susan to the doctor, but at the last minute, she could not take her. So Susan asked her daughter, Linda, for help. Although it was short notice, Linda, who lived on the far side of town, took her mother to the appointment.

Linda asked to sit with her mother during the appointment. The doctor began asking Susan questions about how she was doing, what she was eating, if she was taking her medications, and if she was getting exercise. Susan's responses were fabrications, communicating she had no issues. Linda was astounded. Why would her mom not tell the doctor how she was? Her mom had never lied before!

As the doctor turned to leave, Linda asked to speak with him privately. The doctor agreed, and they stepped out of the room. Linda said her mom's answers were fantasy. Her mom was not doing well on many levels.

The doctor was surprised but turned and went back into the exam room. He told Susan there were some other things he wanted to check. He had her stand and sit several times without using her arms. She walked around the room, closed her eyes while holding her arms out and touching her nose, and other tests. He carefully watched Susan struggle with some of the simple tasks. While watching her, they conversed about her driving, how she got groceries, where the best stores for fresh fruit were, and how expensive fish was. He asked if she was following politics and what was happening at church and so on. He had a different view of his patient after Linda's intervention.

Why was Susan not honest with her physician? There are many answers to this question, though several tend to be more prevalent. The first is caused by the fraternal twins: pride and fear. Older people are proud of their independence. Older people are doing well if they are alone in their homes and taking care of everything. Few, if any of us, want our children or others to think that we are incapable of living at home. It is a matter of pride.

A foundation of that self-sufficiency is fear of loss. Elders sometimes fear their doctors, family members, or others may try to force them out of their homes if they admit frailty at any level. Because of pride and fear, they will fiercely fight any notion that they are not independent. Even seeing a doctor can be a threatening and stressful experience. Having an adult child meeting with the doctor can make some older people even more anxious.

Physicians are tangentially frightening to people in subtle ways. They help their patients by selecting from many different therapies. They might prescribe medications, referrals, therapies; or encourage people to drink more water, eat better food; or at times, prescribe surgery. The cost of medications, referrals, therapy, or other treatments can be frightfully high. Medicare is helpful but hardly pays for full care. When funds are tight, elders must choose between their physician's recommendations and what is affordable.

When the doctor's recommendations are followed, elders must figure out how to get to and from the therapies or how to obtain and pay for medications. Home delivery from pharmacies and home care can help, but transportation can be a huge barrier for elder care, and treatments cost even more. The financial burden of these issues can force elders to choose between necessities and medical care.

Many older people consider their financial situation to be a personal matter, not to be shared outside of the family. When with medical professionals, they can be reticent to reveal that they cannot afford treatment or even that getting to and from various treatments can be arduous. Physicians may ask their elderly patients if they are taking their medications regularly. Elders may be afraid or embarrassed to say that they do not have money for the prescription or that they cut medications in half to conserve them (or share with a spouse). Although alternatives are available to pay for and have medications delivered, elders may be unaware of them or lack the technical know-how to access the information.

Another reason people may not speak to the doctor honestly is that they may not remember, hear, or understand the question and how to answer it. These people have spent sixty years functioning in social settings. And frankly, they are well practiced at being social. After decades of experience, surviving in social environments becomes second nature. One day I spoke with May, a pleasant older woman who had some cognitive decline but was very proper in her questions and responses. As we conversed, I asked about her activities and her favorite foods and recipes. May grew vague the longer we talked. She could not answer questions in detail. She seemed uncomfortable and excused herself to greet a friend a little distance away. She could only respond well so long as the conversation was basic, reflecting common themes experienced through life so her ingrained social skills apply. Yet those skills could not carry May far before she needed to disengage.

Our social skills seem to work similarly to muscle memory. People may not be aware of the situations around them, but their decades-long habits of greeting others and exchanging social pleasantries can remain. This may help explain how a person with serious memory loss may carry on a conversation that, in their minds, is totally cogent while making little sense to the listener.

Here are a few examples of some types of memory loss. A prim and proper lady at church knew all of the hymns by heart. She smiled and nodded at old friends and said hello to all near her. Then she got lost on the way to the restroom.

A man can talk about a type of wood and how hard or soft it is, but he cannot tell you how to get to the shop to buy it.

When asked a question, some people with cognitive decline may create an answer they feel fits the question, though it may not reflect the facts. Alternatively, some older people can tell facts but, for a variety of reasons, cannot express them clearly or at all.

Just because an elder has a memory lapse or forgets a name is not a signal of memory loss. Sometimes these occurrences can happen with those who have no memory loss. I once had a surgeon tell me that I needed surgery on my arm. The office called me several weeks later and asked me when I was going to schedule my surgery. "What surgery?" I asked. I simply did not hear what the doctor had plainly told me. Some studies have suggested people's IQs drop significantly when they become a hospital patient. Older people perceive doctors differently than do younger generations. My point is that nervousness and prior bad experiences alone can contribute to some people answering the doctor's (or others') questions unreliably.

Therefore, most of us would benefit from having an advocate when entering the health system for care. This is particularly true of the frail or people with even a touch of memory loss. What does an advocate look like, and how do adult children and surrogates fit into that advocacy role?

From the broadest possible viewpoint, one might consider the Bible to be one long story of advocacy. The Bible speaks at length and in many ways of God's love and his pursuit of us in both the Old Testament and New Testament. In that love and pursuit, God advocates on our behalf creatively and constantly, even though we may not recognize it. Think about how our next breath draws in air and sustains our lives. God planned and prepared the air and our lungs so we can live. Psalm 19 speaks of the majesty of nature and how it reveals God's providence. More to the point, as the perfect Advocate, he provided us with a plethora of Bible stories showing both his advocacy and how we can be advocates (we are made in his image). His message of advocacy for us, and our advocacy for others, is from cover to cover in the Word of God. God feels so strongly about advocacy that he sent his Son as the perfect Advocate for us, and then he provided us even more support in the Holy Spirit, called the *Paraclete* or the Advocate, to live within us.

The Bible supplies many examples of advocacy, helping us to see and understand the role and various functions of an advocate. Boaz advocated for Ruth and Naomi's welfare and family line. Esther called on King Xerxes to allow Jews to protect themselves. Joseph's birth family was threatened with starvation, so he provided them food, shelter, land, and protection. This was despite his brothers' earlier actions to harm him. Later in history, Pharaoh's daughter rescued the baby Moses from the Nile River. Daniel prayed and fasted so a remnant could return to Israel at the end of the seventy years of captivity. Truly, Jesus is the highest demonstration of advocacy by exchanging his life for ours long before the birth of our generation. In each of our lives, a time will arrive when we are called to be an advocate too. Whether by our choice or not, one of those times is when we need to advocate for an elder.

Advocating for an older person can be tricky. For an elder to thrive today, think about meals, medication, exercise, and socialization as four vital pillars. There are many ways advocates can address these pillars, ensuring the elder's basic needs are met. The first three pillars of meals, medication, and exercise are easy to recognize. The fourth, socialization, is sometimes missed by advocates. The physical and emotional impact of prolonged isolation has huge ramifications on the first three pillars. The classic case is the older widow living on cereal in the morning and tea and toast for supper. Making dinner is often too much work for a person living alone. Isolation tends to attenuate time with few touchpoints for its passing. Hence, older people sometimes over- or under-medicate themselves, especially when living alone. The point is that God created people to live and interact in community with others. Socialization is just that, daily face-to-face interaction with others.

I wondered why my elderly grandmother always wanted to attend church and the women's group even when she could not move or hear well. She had a love of the church and intuitively recognized that she needed to see and spend time with other people, especially her friends. Even introverts need to see and communicate with others. Total lack of socialization (better known as isolation) is detrimental to our health and being.

Couples can also lack socialization. An elder couple may not interact much, and there is something about women being with women and men with men that has different dynamics than spouses together. Elder couples can suffer from a lack of socialization and need outside connections to remain emotionally healthy.

Let's explore a few ways family members can advocate for the elders in their lives.

Juanita, a registered nurse, worried how little her mom, Isabella, was eating and socializing. She began advocating for Isabella by looking for things that would reduce her mother's everyday burdens. Juanita knew that if her husband and children engaged in supporting her mom, they would address many of Isabella's social needs, and Juanita could get easy entry into her mom's pantry. She had her son, Mateo, use his grandmother's lawnmower and care for her lawn without pay. Isabella regularly thanked family and friends by making her special sugar cookies for them. In the fall, the family raked leaves, and in the winter, Mateo and his younger sister shoveled snow and made snow angels in the yard. The grandchildren enjoyed warming up with Isabella's hot chocolate and listening to her stories of when she was a girl. Isabella appreciated these simple acts of kindness, and the relationships with the grandchildren deepened.

Juanita supported her mother by dropping in to visit, "just happening" to swing by the grocery store first. She would bring along an item or two she knew her mom would like. That allowed Juanita to look into Isabella's refrigerator and cupboards to see what was there. She then jotted down needed items and planned to make some meals with her mother.

On her next visit, Juanita brought something else her mom needed and liked. Eventually, Juanita could figure out what her mom was using. This way, she was assured that her mom was cooking and eating, and Isabella benefited from family socialization. And because she was regularly in the house, Juanita could keep an eye on its state of repair. If something needed to be fixed, she quietly helped make that happen.

Harriet knew that traffic would be bad when her dad, Elijah, had his medical appointments, so she drove him there. Then she began going into the treatment room with her dad and asking relevant questions. Harriet even took short notes of what the doctor said so she and her dad could keep the instructions straight. As Elijah grew forgetful at the doctor's questions, she cued him or said things like, "Didn't you say you were having…" Harriet was wise not to answer for her dad because he would have taken it as an affront to his independence.

Miriam's three daughters, Julie, Sandy, and Amy, all lived several hundred miles from their childhood home. Miriam had raised her daughters and loved her husband in that house. As time passed her three daughters grew up and moved to jobs in other states. Miriam was comfortable and always loved her home of forty-seven years. Sadly, she began experiencing memory loss and needed caregivers to help with meals and bathing. The daughters were worried and together created a plan to look after their mom. For several years, the daughters created a rotation in which each stayed with their mom for a week to ten days.

The daughter staying with Miriam took care of her needs, ensuring the caregivers were properly attending to her. When staying with their mom, the daughters used their mom's car and drove her to the hairdresser, the pharmacy, the doctor, and other appointments. Because the time commitment was high, they usually let a week or two pass between the time one daughter left and the next arrived.

Julie, Sandy, and Amy held a conference call following each one's visit. They discussed how the time went with Miriam and if any of their plans needed revising due to her slow decline. They did not want to move her from her home because she was comfortable there and felt safe. Her anxiety and memory loss were worsened whenever she was out of her home for more than an hour or two. During one visit, Julie gave emergency phone numbers with pictures of her mom to neighbors and the local police in case her mother got turned around in the neighborhood.

The three sisters advocated in a way many families cannot. However, in executing their plan, they each gained personal experience with their mom, communicated often about what was happening, and together planned for their mom's care.

Often, a distant family member who is not seeing the day-to-day experience of an older person has great difficulty in understanding the challenges of the current situation. The reality is fully grasped only by personal ongoing presence. Miriam's daughters avoided much of the conflict families have with some of the participants/decision makers who cannot see the day-to-day realities because of distance. There are times that families in conflict need to take a break and say, "This is hard. Let's not make a decision right now. Instead, let's sit down and just talk."

However, some older people do not think they need an advocate. What then?

People like to remain in control of their lives and are resistant to help. "Oh, no, honey, I'll do that tomorrow." And then conveniently forget to do whatever "it" was. Another issue is when an elder or elder couple refuses to see that any change is needed. They become entrenched in their lifestyles regardless of the less-than-optimum quality they may be experiencing.

Maria was so convinced she needed no help that she fired every caregiver her children sent to her apartment. Yet she expected and demanded aid from next-door neighbors, friends, and the ambulance crews. Maria was incapable of seeing her situation for what it was.

These situations sometimes require a family intervention, using the physician, police (regarding driving), or adult protective services if necessary—a serious and messy confrontation. Sad as it is, it might be the only way to surround older people with the needed help so that they can thrive. At times, the refusal to accept help or move to a supportive environment is irrational, possibly caused by the fraternal twins' pride and fear. Or consider that it might be cognitive decline, and they are unable to think well of their situation.

In cognitive decline, setting up a power of attorney (POA) may not be particularly helpful because the POA must be signed while the person is still rational. If someone is incapable of making decisions, a Durable POA for Health Care may be proper. However, the only way to legally ensure an elder does not make decisions for himself is to go to court and have him deemed incompetent. (Most people rely on the POA as all they need to move their parents. But be aware of possible limitations.)

Forcing a difficult situation with interventions could be necessary and doable, though painful. Until someone is considered legally incompetent, he can make his own decisions regardless of what others believe about him. Mark and John were concerned that their father, Bill, was refusing to leave his house and dog. Bill was not eating well, and he cut his medicines in half to save money. He did not care well for the dog. Bill had several handguns and said that he did not want his sons to force him into an assisted living. Bill told them that he would choose death over an institution. Bill's out-of-control blood pressure was exacerbated by his habit of cutting pills in half to save money. One day he was dizzy and fell sideways onto his hip in the bathroom, which required surgery and recovery in a nursing home's rehab center. While being taken out of his home was not a preferred outcome for Bill, Mark and John arranged for Bill's move to an assisted living. John took the dog into his home after promising Bill to have the dog visit him weekly.

In situations where an elder refuses to comply with reason, the advocate remains proactive in unexpected ways. Rather than argue with her parents, the advocate can do all in her power to make the living environment safe and healthy. The advocate can register the elders for Meals on Wheels, for example. The advocate might get into the home and remove slip and trip hazards or install night-lights or even home cameras (with the elder's permission). The other action of the advocate is to think through various scenarios that might occur and have a plan prepared in those circumstances.

Chris's parents lived several states distant from him. From spending time with them earlier that year, he recognized that they had some memory loss. He saw firsthand how they were struggling with food, transportation, medications, and daily life. He tried, unsuccessfully, to convince his parents to move closer to either his sister, Susan, or him. His mother called him one day asking if he would ask Susan to stop over and help them take care of a few things around the house. Chris said, "Mom, you remember Susan lives eight hours away from you. She cannot come over and fix you a meal or take care of a few things today. It is too far." Shortly after that conversation, Chris's parents asked their children's help in finding a rental house near Susan. Chris and Susan's hopes to help their parents came to fruition only when the parents could fully realize the difficulty of their situation. Chris's honesty with his mother helped break through to a solution.

A couple lived in a rural home. They ate who-knew-what and lived in deplorable conditions. Michael loved his parents and tried to intervene, but they refused to move or to receive any support. He thought his dad, Ray, was emotionally forcing his wife, Katherine, to be his caregiver. Katherine agreed to care for her husband because she had vowed "for better or worse." But Katherine needed surgery, and Ray could not stay alone due to the medication and personal care he needed. It was not a happy situation, but Michael helped Katherine convince Ray to go to an assisted living center at least while she was in the hospital and recovering after surgery. It worked. After her recovery, Michael helped his mom understand that caring for Ray was causing her to fail. After several long talks and many tears, Katherine and Michael decided that the best for both parents would be for Dad to remain in the assisted living center. Katherine later moved into the assisted living to be near Ray.

Edwardo and Sophia had never spent a night apart in their sixty-two years of marriage. Sophia had severe memory loss. Edwardo decided that since they did not have children, it would be best if they moved together into a mid-priced retirement community with small homes. The retirement community's admission counselor asked Edwardo about his emergency plans for Sophia if something happened to him. Edwardo was defensive, saying that they had always been together and would remain that way.

Two weeks before they moved into their new home, Edwardo came down with the flu that led to pneumonia and had to be hospitalized. Both Edwardo and Sophia were in trouble. Though ill, Edwardo called the admissions counselor to see if Sophia could move into one of the care areas until he recovered. The retirement community helped move Sophia to their Memory Care area temporarily. Edwardo moved into the retirement community's rehab program and then to the assisted living center until he fully recovered, about seven months later.

Upon his recovery, he decided that moving Sophia to another place on the campus would be too overwhelming for her. He admitted that he probably caught the flu because he was not caring well enough for himself. He conceded that he could better supply love and support for Sophia while she was in the Memory Care area. It was better that she remained there rather than bring her home with him.

When an elder is in a hospital for a major health event like a fractured hip or surgery, she often follows her hospital stay with rehabilitation in a nursing home. This can be a short stay of a few weeks. If an advocate senses the elder needs more support than she can get at home, the advocate can engage the attending physicians, social workers, and case managers with open and frank discussions of the concerns and ask for help with meeting the needs. An advocate will seldom have more support and options for communicating a temporary or permanent change than when an elder is in the hospital. If an advocate thinks ahead, he may have quietly scoped out nursing homes and assisted livings in advance as a "just in case" plan should it be needed.

Hospitals encourage short stays and will often not give much notice, saying something like, "Your mom needs to be discharged to a nursing home for therapy in two days. Where do you want her to go?" The advocate needs to consider the next desired placement in advance rather than be rushed into a decision without much information. Advocates plan for the best possible decisions for the elder should an emergency occur.

Another technique for helping elders who refuse to honestly face their situations is to reframe the conversation with possibilities they are not considering. Jermain had a conversation with his reluctant father, Curtis, about handling bills. "Dad, a lot of other people unexpectedly end up in the hospital. I hope that never happens to you. But if that were to happen to you, what do you think you might need? Paying the bills on time is important to you, but I do not want to go rooting through your personal things. So not to intrude, can you show me where you keep your important papers?" A little further into the conversation, Jermain said, "Dad, heaven forbid, but sometimes people are in a hospital and then have to go to a rehab center. How would your bills get paid during that time? Just in an emergency, how would I know what to do? I could write checks and bring the checks to you to sign. Or if it would make it easier for you, you could permit me to pay bills on your behalf as your POA—but only when you allow."

When an advocate arrives on the scene, people (old or not!) often assume the advocate has an agenda that is not in the elder's favor. "You're here to move me out of my house!" Or "You want me to live with your sister, and I'm not leaving my friends." Or even, "You're here to take me to the nursing home!" This can lead to incorrect assumptions and issues that would be better to step around. As an advocate, do not start with either a hidden agenda or promises you may not be able to keep. Instead, consider how Joseph in the Bible asked pointed questions of his brothers and listened closely to what was said and not said. He also took time to observe how they behaved toward one another so he could meaningfully respond to their needs.

Often the discussion about the Living Will and Durable Power of Attorney for Health Care is uncomfortable. Approach the subject matter-of-factly. "I want you to be healthy and live long, but we do not know God's plans for us. Frankly, none of us in the family want to guess your wishes in the worst-case scenario. The doctor will not guess either. If we put your wishes in writing, we can give a copy to your doctor. Then in case of an emergency, you will get the medical treatment in the way you want."

Many states have a specific form to use. An internet search should produce those documents. Usually, a lawyer is not needed for this document.

The Durable Power of Attorney for Health Care (DPOAH) is used in case the elder is incapacitated and temporarily cannot make a vital health-care decision. The DPOH is in effect only when the person is incapacitated, which can mean unconscious, in a comatose state, or deemed legally incompetent by a court. The elder chooses who will represent him or her.

Both the Living Will and DPOAH are critically important in the worst-case situations. More than one family has agonized over decisions about their permanently incapacitated loved ones whose future meaningful lives are limited.

Four adult children had to face the decision of having their father's ventilator turned off. They did not know his specific wishes because they had never discussed them with him. They spoke with the doctor and prayed. Then they made a decision based on what they thought their father would want. Before they could inform the social worker, the doctor came into the room where they were deliberating and said that their father's condition had improved and they would be able to remove the breathing tube.

The discussion about these things with the elder can be hard but not as hard as being in a situation where a decision must be made with no guidance from the individual. None of these children ever forgot the difficulty of that heart-wrenching decision.

The Role of Technology

My grandmother raised her five children on a farm in South Dakota. They had pioneered on the land, their home built by my grandfather. When I stayed there with my family, my grandmother cooked meals on a wood-burning stove. She used a special handle to lift the round cast-iron tops off the stove to make sure the fire under that area of the stove or oven was exactly right. A huge technological advancement for her was when she moved into a small house in town and bought a harvest gold electric stove; however, it took time and practice before she could cook well on that new stove.

The point is that technology can help people stay independent longer. It is simply a tool that advocates can use to aid and protect their loved ones. The electric stove enabled my grandmother to stay independent longer because she could not chop wood any longer, and carrying and stowing the wood was burdensome.

Technology has prerequisites to work properly, and they will need reliable, safe help for using any meaningful technology. Typically, some source of electricity is needed as well as a connection through cellular service, phone lines, or an internet signal. The complexity of setting up Wi-Fi networks and connecting devices is daunting for some older people and impossible for others.

Some of the earliest technologies were home alarm systems and emergency call devices. Those systems have advanced into wireless signal and Wi-Fi tools with video service, locking devices, and motion sensors. Cellular phones have features that allow parents to track their children when they are away from home. The same types of applications can work well for adult children to follow their parents' travels. The near-instant communications do not need much discussion here because they are common and available. The issue is helping older people learn to use technology.

If an older person becomes frail, forgetful, or wanders, helpful technologies are available. As above, using the systems that have motion sensors and camera views can aid in keeping an eye on an elder. If wandering is an issue, the appropriate technology can alert a family member that elopement is occurring and the direction the person went. Installing automatic locks on doors and motion sensor cameras can alert family members when a person leaves the home. GPS tracking devices can be placed on cars. Wi-Fi accessible thermostats can help ensure comfortable temperatures are maintained. Watches with tracking devices can be worn or attached to devices like walkers or canes. In the field of elder services, providers used to unplug stoves and, sometimes, microwaves. That still works, but timers might be more helpful.

All these tools are part of the "internet of things" and will be most useful as the companies gather data on older people's needs. Companies are developing fall monitors that capture an elder's walking gate. As an example, one company has enough data from their fall systems that, using artificial intelligence and sophisticated algorithms, they can predict with high confidence that an elder will likely have a fall before it occurs.

More helpful tools are available, or will be in the future, such as automatic pill dispensers that ensure the right person takes the right dose at the right time. If a dose is overlooked, the machine will contact someone to check on the elder. Watches and other devices are available that help monitor sleep, weight, blood sugar levels, and blood pressure. All of these can be helpful for adult children to watch after their older parents, particularly if the parent has comorbidity such as diabetes, congestive heart failure, or other common issues.

The key to these tools is to make them simple to use. Older people are entirely capable of learning how to use technology. However, some have limited eyesight, hearing, and touch and taste sensations, all of which challenge the learning process. The loss of recent memory (caused by many different factors—some that can be addressed) can further impede an elder's ability to learn to use a technological tool. Childlike simplicity can be demeaning as can advertising aimed at "old people." Look for technology that is reliable, simple, and adult in presentation.

Besides simple operation features, another important element in using technology is motivating the elder to use it. My grandmother's harvest gold electric stove was simple to use. Knowing that it would help her remain independent was her motivation to learn how to use it. Learning to use technology to keep family connected and elders independent is important. Help the older person understand that using technology keeps them independent. Although the older person may believe he is safe, the safety benefit of the device(s) may be more assuring to the adult child than to the parent.

Application

In simplest terms, the role of an advocate is to consider another person's interests as more important than the advocate's. It sounds much like Paul's admonishment in Philippians 2:4, "Rather in humility value others above yourselves, not looking to your own interests but each of you to the interests of the others." The hard part of advocacy is getting out of your own way and trying to understand the perspective and experience of the elder. To succeed in this, advocates must carefully watch and walk alongside the elders. Avoid the temptation to muscle into the elder's life and give solutions you think are right before listening to the older person and understanding what she needs for her best life. We all define what we think is best for us and that perspective does not change just because we get older.

Advocating for others is challenging because of their thoughts and desires, their self-perception of their ability and situation, health as well as cognitive changes. Isaac Newton's First Law of Motion is that an object will not change its motion until acted upon by another force. Each life has a certain trajectory from the sum of our decisions and experiences. The advocate must step inside the elder's trajectory and be the guiding force for the elder's safety, security, health, and dignity. There is no easy answer for elders refusing or unable to objectively appraise their own circumstances. The first order of the advocate is to support and develop a relationship with the older person for trust and assurance. There will be conflict, but in the context of trust, the advocate can be the best expression of the elder's choices and desires.

Takeaway Thoughts

The way God structured the Jewish law and culture and sent Jesus to us are two examples proving how he loves and advocates for us. God places us in positions to advocate for others. Following God's example, the act of advocacy is an act of compassion. There are few accolades or medals for being an advocate, at least on this side of heaven. We do not often consider the nobility and honor of the elder's advocate's acts of self-sacrifice. Yet it is a high aspiration to advocate well, following in the footsteps of God.

Questions for Consideration

1. This chapter suggested several times when an advocate stepped forward in the Bible. Describe other examples of advocacy from the Bible.

2. Think of a time when someone was an advocate for you. How did you respond?
3. Have you been called on to advocate for a person? How were you able to think of his or her interests as more important than your own in that situation?
4. How would you begin to advocate for an older person in your life?
5. In what ways can you use technology to help an elder meet his or her needs?
6. Pick one of the examples of advocacy in this chapter. Do you agree or disagree with how that situation was handled? Why or why not? What would you do differently, given the same circumstances?

5

Presentation of Aging Challenges

President Reagan's verbal sparring while debating Senator Mondale revealed our culture's fear of aging—that a time might come when we are too old to matter. As gifted and strong as Reagan was, there may have been signs during his second term, shadowed glimpses, of the future Alzheimer's disease that would eventually claim his memory and self. As gifts and experiences morph lives over time, we are confronted with the question drawn by corruption: What happens when aging becomes problematic?

Six men gathered early one morning at a local restaurant a few days before Good Friday. With Bibles in one hand and cups of coffee in the other, they discussed the humanity and divinity of Jesus and how he had come to fulfill the law and prophets (Matt. 5:17).

One of the men said that he had landed on the word *fulfill* in the verse and spent some time looking at the word's meaning in the original language. Scholars generally said it could be translated as "complete," "fulfilled," "perfected," or "the final step." One scholar clarified it further. His point was that as soon as God uttered a word, it was true from that moment in time and place. The word in the original Greek usually translated as "fulfilled" also means "to fulfill a demand or claim," i.e., "for something stated in the past to be entirely completed, actualized, carried out, executed, or accomplished." A modern example may be that when a house is purchased, ownership passes to the buyer on the date of the closing. The new owner pays the mortgage and taxes from that point. However, often the new owner cannot take possession until a future date. My wife and I had to wait a month before we could move into one house we had purchased. In our case, the legal agreement happened on one day, but the agreement was not fully complete (fulfilled) until we moved in and took possession. In Matthew 5:17, Jesus said he came to fulfill (fully complete) the law and prophets.

Then one view of the Old Testament is as a picture, blueprint, or promise of New Testament reality (fulfillment). (See Hebrews 10:1–2, Romans 15:4, 1 Corinthians 10:6–11.) Jesus is our Savior and the author of our faith while also the example as the firstborn Son of God. He ushered in the kingdom of God and placed his Holy Spirit within us to live as "Ambassadors"—the same word as "elders."

In the Bible study mentioned above, one man, John, commented that an ambassador carries the authority, strength, and voice of the country he or she represents. Another man, Gordon, pointed out that the title of the ambassador is Mr./Madam Ambassador or Ambassador (last name). Ambassadors can create respect for their home country simply by how they carry themselves and work with others in the foreign land. In the context of the study, the men challenged one another to be ambassadors of God of the highest order and to live distinguished lives, bringing honor to the kingdom of God.

Assuming the above is correct, the first four chapters of this book have shown us that (1) God designed us to live and age in the context of community, and (2) God was not surprised by our great corruption. Not only did he give us redemption through Jesus but also, in his boundless compassion, he structured families, clans, and tribes to protect the weak and vulnerable. Then he created law based on his presence and compassion in such a way to ensure the frail and vulnerable would have a respected place in society and that if impoverished, they would have support to rebuild their lives. The attitudes and language he calls us to use with the aging and poor are borne of deep respect, thoughtfulness, and compassion. Then to the aging, God bestows special gifts and attributes. Together, all of these components are foundational tools for use in apprehending (fulfilling) our own aging and lifting those who go before us.

Taking from the lesson of the men's Bible study, we understand that God laid out a blueprint for not only how we are to treat one another but also, more specifically, how we are to regard and treat the aging, frail, and poor. As ambassadors of God's goodwill toward people precious to him, we are imperfect. But God has designed us and impelled us by the Holy Spirit to work with one another as we address the results of the great corruption in one another.

The balance of this book provides perspectives and examples of how using God's design may help inform and instruct us in carrying out and actualizing his compassion and plan for ourselves and the aging today. Jesus commanded us to love one another, and it is our purpose now to fulfill (make complete) that truth in one another's lives.

Continuous Transition

"You could not step twice into the same river; for new waters are ever flowing on to you" (Heraclitus of Ephesus).

As in the flow of a river, each of life's moments is a transition to the next. As adults, we tend to see life in a semipermanent way. Change occurs in our lives almost imperceptibly, and years pass almost undetectably until we suddenly look back to see how much has gone. We celebrate certain milestones to help us recognize the transitions: confirmations, graduations, first jobs, marriage, and so on. Yet each period of life sees us transition in our physical, financial, relational, mental, spiritual, and emotional selves, with each aspect essential and central to our future lives and experiences. In this sense, our lives are compounded, each phase building on the previous one.

However, unlike the river, as we pass through each stage, we never leave all the former times completely behind. Like sticky resin from tree sap, memories, events, and relationships stay with us from the day they occur until we take them to death. And like revisionist historians, our understanding of and the meaning we ascribe those memories can subtly change in the context of new knowledge and experience.

This growth or maturation is one reason we can never go back and fully reexperience the past. This is also one way we each become more uniquely "ourselves" as we age. In this sense we are always transitioning to becoming more ourselves. Every decision we make helps define and create who we will be in the future, especially those choices we repeat that become habitual choices. Those things we learn and the perspectives we adopt deeply affect how we understand and experience the physical, financial, relational, mental, spiritual, and emotional aspects of life as we age. In each of these, we are laying the foundation that undergirds successes and failures in aging for ourselves and those close to us.

Comorbidity: Multiple Health Issues

Comorbidity is the fancy term for having more than one illness at a time. Typically, the term relates to chronic issues such as diabetes, chronic obstructive pulmonary disease (COPD), ongoing heart disease, or other disorders. Usually, it relates to serious health conditions more than high blood pressure or sleep apnea. It is common as we age to have more than one chronic condition at a time.

As older people age, it is common to experience comorbidity. Diabetes seems to spawn multiple other conditions. Comorbidities challenge health professionals. Rather than having cures for most chronic diseases, health professionals help their patients manage the disease, typically through medications. Medications have a variety of side effects. As the number of conditions increases, the potential for medication side effects increases. Medication for one condition may cause nausea, for which another medication might be prescribed. Rather than being an indictment of prescription medicines, this points to a serious concern for elders: polypharmacy, when multiple medications are needed for an individual to manage disorders. Three main concerns arise with polypharmacy.

The first is older people may have more than one physician or health practitioner prescribing medication for them. If a physician does not know about all medications and supplements a person takes, an elder can easily take too much of one that counteracts others. Either case can be life threatening.

The second concern is adherence to the times and dosages of medications. Younger people can usually miss taking a dose of a prescription with little ill effect. Elders have more challenges. "Researchers estimate that 25 percent of people ages 65 to 69 take at least five prescription drugs to treat chronic conditions, a figure that jumps to nearly 46 percent for those between 70 and 79. Doctors say it is not uncommon to encounter patients taking more than 20 drugs to treat acid reflux, heart disease, depression or insomnia or other disorders."[1]

Medication errors by seniors are common. Imagine taking five or ten different medications for multiple disorders or symptoms. Each prescription has a proper time and application. Each bottle has a label with fine print. Elders often have a hard time seeing and even matriculating the pills due to size, limitation of hand movement, or finger sensation. Then some of the pills are to be taken before meals, others after, some between meals, and some before bedtime or first thing in the morning. The plethora of medications can be so confusing long-term care organizations use sophisticated electronic medical records to keep it straight for everyone. Pharmacists are required to periodically review the medication record with computerized systems to ensure the medications do not interact.

A son noticed his mom's decline and knew the retirement community she lived in had a nurse available for residents who lived independently. It seemed to him that his mom was beginning not to think or and speak as cogently as she had. She had dropped out of several social groups she previously enjoyed. He contacted the nurse, who visited his mother. During the visit, the nurse mentioned she had not seen the elder woman attending as many groups and events as before and asked if she was experiencing some challenges.

"I don't have any energy. I talked with my doctor about it, but nothing is improving," the woman said.

May I look at the medicines you are taking?" the nurse asked.

The elder collected her medicines.

The nurse spread out the multiple bottles on a table and asked if the medicines were all taken daily. Then reading the bottle labels and listing the medicines, she noted that they were from different pharmacies and that several doctors were prescribing the same or similar medicines to the woman. She also noted a potentially life-threatening contraindication between two of the medicines. The nurse, together with the woman, called the doctors and made necessary medication changes. She also helped the woman to move all her medications to a single pharmacy, thus avoiding medication duplication and saving the woman money. Not many days later the older woman reappeared at social gatherings and clubs and her energy returned.

Finally, too often elders cannot afford their medications. It is well known that due to cost, expensive prescriptions are either not purchased or not used in keeping with the instructions. According to Senator Grassley's website,

> [There] is a rising percentage of adults who report not having had enough money in the past 12 months to 'pay for needed medicine or drugs that a doctor prescribed' to them. This percentage has increased significantly, from 18.9% in January 2019 to 22.9% in September. In all, the 22.9% represents about 58 million adults who experienced 'medication insecurity,' defined as the inability to pay for prescribed medication at least one time in the past 12 months.[2]

The elderly and others with limited incomes often cannot afford the medications they need. Therefore, they may go without the medicine or decrease the amount they take (e.g., cut the pill in half).

A Leading Cause of Elder Injury and Death

Someone once said that life is dangerous because it always ends in a terminal event. While this is true, well-known reasons lead to that terminal event: heart disease, stroke, cancer...the list goes on.

An unexpected "terminal event" is related to falls. Certainly, the fall itself can be deadly for an older person. I heard of an older woman who died from a fall. She lost her balance, and as she fell to the floor, her head hit the corner of a coffee table.

Most fall-related deaths tend to occur from complications of the fall. There is about a 70 percent mortality rate within a year of older people who have major surgery because of a fall. The trauma of the fall, surgery, sudden life change, financial strain, and recovery process add up and exacerbate underlying conditions. The person's death might be from another direct cause—such as a stroke or heart attack—but the direct cause of death can often be traced back to a traumatic fall.

The question to ask is, how often do adults between their twenties and fifties fall? It is not common. Should we expect people in their sixties, seventies, and beyond to fall? Why do older people fall?

Elder falls occur from a combination of factors that can be cumulative. Often a critical part of the fall is due to loss of strength and balance. Physical and occupational therapy, which a physician can order, are important tools for older people to retain strength and balance. Or an older person can use a program, a trainer, or even television or internet trainers to stay strong and help avoid falls. Older people can build muscle mass into their late nineties with proper nutrition and training.

Other reasons for falls are poor eyesight, trip hazards, inadequate lighting, medications, and alcohol. It is critical to go through an elder's home and remove scatter rugs, old slippers with holes, and furniture or other items encroaching on a walking path. Any plumbing or equipment that leaks needs to be repaired or replaced. Nightlights illuminating the walking path to the bathroom and kitchen are vital. Installing a motion-activated light in the bathroom can be effective, especially if it does not turn on full, bright lights suddenly, which can contribute to a fall. Dim lights or a light that starts dim and slowly brightens is much better.

A high percentage of falls occur in the bathroom. Providing safe handrails, using a shower, or helping an elder in and out of the tub can be effective in preventing falls. The bathroom is especially bad because it usually is a confined space with many hard and even wet (slippery) surfaces. If possible, use a nonslip floor surface in the bathroom. Place anti-slip mats in tubs and showers. Add a shower or bath chair so an elder can sit down while bathing or showering. Make sure towel bars are easily reached from the tub or shower (without having to stretch for them). Use only unbreakable items in the bathroom (including decorative items). Have shampoo and body wash mounted on the wall of the shower stall so that the bottles cannot be dropped (ensure the dispensers do not leak). Store frequently used items in easily reached areas so the elder does not have to bend or search for them. The financial cost to repair a broken bone from a fall is high, especially if major surgery and rehabilitation are needed. It is a good investment to make the home safe than to endure the physical, emotional, and financial cost of a fall.

Investigate the cause of a fall even if there is no apparent injury. When a person has multiple falls over a few days or weeks, it is often an indication that something has changed and needs attention. It is better to visit the doctor than to end up in an emergency room with a major issue. It is important to see a physician to review what could medically contribute to a fall. The doctor can refer helpful therapies to build strength and balance. It is embarrassing to fall, and commonly an elder will not mention the fall. So family members should be watchful for unexplained bruises or sores that might be fall related and get assistance to prevent further falls.

A family member once told an admissions counselor that they were bringing their mother to the assisted living because she was falling too often. The staff member asked if they had visited the doctor to help understand the cause of the falls.

"No, why?" the family member answered.

"It is important to address the cause for falls. No senior care service can promise that an elder will not fall," the staff member answered.

Even if a person has constant personal care and multiple preventive steps, falls will still occur. Identifying the cause can reduce the risk of another fall and avoid issues down the road. (See Resources for additional information on falls.)

Physical Foundations

After briefly touching on health, nutrition, and exercise, we will turn to several frequent aspects of physical aging that are important but often overlooked in other discussions. The information I provide is not intended as medical advice and is intentionally incomplete. I am not a physician or clinical practitioner.

Since the Scriptures declare that each of our days is measured out for us, it makes sense to maximize the quality of life we experience in each of those days. Eating a healthy diet, ensuring quality medical care, participating in meaningful socialization, and getting regular exercise are key to maintaining our best level of health. The time to start is now.

Landmark research from the 1980s proved that people even older than ninety could develop muscle mass if they had healthy nutrition and appropriate exercise. Regaining strength and balance is possible (within limits and a physician's support) unless a specific disease process is at work inhibiting growth. Start the process by discussing it with the elder's physician. Look for a reasonable, appropriate, and safe plan for nutrition and exercise, and stick to it as a daily habit. Variety is needed to keep it fresh. It is even easier to stick to a plan when like-minded friends are also involved. If you enjoy a particular physical activity but can no longer do it, look for ways to modify the activity. Maintaining physical levels of activity positively affects every other aspect of life.

Nursing homes demonstrated that once people sit down in a wheelchair for "convenience," they often remain in it for the balance of their lives, even if they were walking routinely before. The convenience issue in nursing homes is caused because, on admission, the elder is simply not strong enough to walk the distance to the dining or bathing rooms without resting (they have not retained their strength). Elders often do not walk much at home or in the hospital, thereby losing strength and balance. Much sedentary time makes people easily tired. Nursing home staff typically do not want the elder to be overtired and unable to eat; therefore, they assist the elder with a wheelchair. Many elders land in a wheelchair within the first twenty-four hours of arriving at a nursing home—often with good intent.

Please note that this experience relates mostly to people who are moving permanently into a nursing home. Many people go to nursing homes for rehabilitation after a fall, surgery, or some other event. These elders intend only a short stay before returning to their former homes. They may need to be in a wheelchair for assistance precisely because they need therapy to rebuild their strength. The key is to ask why an elder may need (or is in) a wheelchair and determine what can be done to maintain and build their strength and balance to get them out of the wheelchair.

Research suggests that the body's physical abilities slow as we age. This is true with physical reaction time as well. Some of this is due to the changes in muscle structure as we age. Whether this is also affected by a slowdown of mental abilities or some other factor, such as the connection between our minds and bodies is slowing, it is not clear. However, our culture today tells us to slow down, chill out, and take a break. Life is too fast-paced, and the speed without control itself causes stress. The gradual slowing of our processes may be a natural way to deal with stress. Being more easily tired might be forcing us to be intentional and purpose driven. This could be a gift to the aging but may also help explain why some elders become more engaged, patient, and magnanimous in their aging years (e.g., think of wonderful grandparents who engage their families warmly regardless of physical limitations). Does this physical slowing create an opportunity for greater personal intentionality? Since research also suggests that active lives tend to stay more active, is "slowing down" a function of a sedentary lifestyle? The answer is likely a little of both.

So how do the Scriptures relate to nutrition, exercise, and socialization? (Socialization was discussed in chapter 4.) After all, Paul advised Timothy, "Have nothing to do with old wives' tales; rather train yourself to be godly. For physical training is of some value, but godliness has value for all things, holding promise for this life and the life to come" (1 Tim. 4:7–8). Contextually, this passage is about ensuring proper doctrine and spiritual training, both necessary to promote godliness. Paul does use the physical training image later in the book to describe how we ought to train ourselves to run the race of faith.

Are the Scriptures silent on the physical disciplines that add to our years? The Scriptures are the inspired Word of God, and in them God does not ignore our need for nutrition, socialization, and exercise. In the times of the Old and New Testaments, walking was the primary mode of transportation. Often, people walked carrying things like buckets of water, produce, or farm loads. Each of their days involved significant manual work. Numerous stories and parables relate to growing, planting, reaping, and fishing, all of which imply physically demanding work. All the carrying and lifting equates to weight training and daily walking. Exercise was implicitly necessary for daily life. Whether living in the country or towns, people did a considerable amount of walking. Physical labor marked each day.

"In older adults, walking below minimum recommended levels is associated with lower all-cause mortality compared with inactivity. Walking at or above physical activity recommendations is associated with even greater decreased risk." [3]

By the nature of the times in which the Bible was written, all of the food was organic. In the structure of agrarian culture, communities of people often worked together to share common tasks and resources. The necessities of each day sufficiently describe the exercise, nutrition, and socialization needed for quality aging.

I grew up in a Minnesota farming community. I served as an orderly in the local hospital and saw firsthand the strength and resilience of the lifelong farm families and the incredible physical strength of the "old Norwegian farmers" from that area. They worked hard, ate what they grew on the farm, and were generous with their time helping and being "neighborly." They were church-going people. They reveal how physical work through a lifetime of eating home-grown nutrition (albeit with quantities of red meat, butter, lard, and cream) and regular socialization added vitality and purpose to their lives.

Today, in postmodern life, exercise, nutrition, and socialization are not requisite to our daily experience; however, they are vital to a healthy life. To get those critical elements, we must thoughtfully introduce them as "additions" to our lives.

How Many People Have Significant Independent Living Limitations?

What happens, though, when physical limitations cause restrictions? A 2016 US Census Bureau report of the American Community Survey discusses many aspects of the US population, including rates of disability among the elderly by age group. The study reviewed disability of six key activities of daily living: vision, hearing, ambulatory (serious difficulty walking or climbing stairs), cognitive (difficulty concentrating, remembering or making decisions), self-care (dressing or bathing), and independent living (difficulty doing errands alone).

> Serious difficulty walking or climbing stairs was the most prevalent disability for all older population age groups. Over 15 percent of those aged 65 to 74 had ambulatory difficulty, along with over a quarter of those aged 75 to 84 and almost half of those 85 and older… The percentage of people with an independent living disability had one of the most noticeable increases: the disability rate for those aged 85 and older was almost six times the rate of those aged 65 to 74.[4]

One of the greatest predictors of an elder moving permanently to a nursing home is the absence of a primary caregiver in the elder's home. And the typical reasons those people move to the nursing home are mobility issues, bowel and bladder incontinence or memory issues with which they need help and support.

It is common for an aging person with physical limitations to have an "event" that causes them to go to a hospital. Professional health and social assessments in the hospital reveal they need twenty-four-hour care or supervision, and "the conversation" occurs. The next step after the hospital is assisted living or the nursing home for rehabilitation and then, possibly, long-term care. Many assisted living centers have criteria that when an elder is no longer continent of bowel and bladder and needs daily assistance with those functions, they are required to move to a nursing home.

The number of elders living in nursing homes is large. But factually, what is the percentage of people who live in nursing homes? Dr. Nancy Wellman, a retired professor of dietetics and nutrition in the Stempel School of Public Health at Florida International University and the former director of the National Resource Center on Nutrition, Physical Activity and Aging, stated at the 2010 Institute of Medicine (US) Food Forum that

> most Americans over the age of 65 live in the community, not in nursing homes or other institutions. Only 4.5 percent (about 1.5 million) of older adults live in nursing homes and 2 percent (1 million) in assisted living facilities. The majority of older adults (93.5 percent, or 33.4 million) live in the community. In fact, she remarked that it is U.S. federal policy to keep people out of nursing homes and to move people who currently live in nursing homes out of nursing homes, partly for budgetary reasons.[5]

While this data is from 2010, it still aptly describes the current environment in which nursing homes are the absolute last desired choice for most elders and their families. Most elders do not live in nursing homes or other institutional environments such as assisted living or congregate living.

> Nearly one-half of older adults, or 18 million people, had difficulty or received help in the last month with daily activities. Altogether, 1 in 4 older adults receiving help lived in either a supportive care (15%) or a nursing home (10%) setting. Nearly 3 million received assistance with

3 or more self-care or mobility activities in set-tings other than nursing homes, and a dispro-portionate share of persons at this level had low incomes. Nearly all older adults in settings other than nursing homes had at least 1 potential infor-mal care network member (family or household member or close friend), and the average num-ber of network members was 4. Levels of infor-mal assistance, primarily from family caregivers, were substantial for older adults receiving help in the community (164 hours/month) and liv-ing in supportive care settings (50 hours/month). Nearly all of those getting help received infor-mal care, and about 3 in 10 received paid care. Of those who had difficulty or received help in settings other than nursing homes, 32% had an adverse consequence in the last month related to an unmet need; for community residents with a paid caregiver, the figure was nearly 60%.[6]

This means that more people are living at home with multi-ple chronic conditions that affect their independence (and families) than live in either a nursing home or other supportive living envi-ronment. The 2020 census shows an increasing number and percent of older people whose activities of daily living or mobility is limited in the US. This is likely because more options for treatment and care of chronic condition are available today and that many towns offer more personal care services.

The elder's home itself may become a physical challenge to healthy and safe living. When an elder's home is on multiple levels, it may become difficult and dangerous to navigate the stairs. As we age, most elders need more lumens of quality light to see adequately; therefore, brighter natural-spectrum bulbs are recommended. Door frames in American homes are often not wide enough to accommo-date a walker or wheelchair and become trip hazards. Many older homes do not have accessible showers or well-placed grab bars. It is important to keep in mind that falls (particularly those in bathrooms) are a huge risk for elders and, as discussed earlier in this chapter, avoiding or stopping them is crucial. For those who have lived in the same home for decades, the heating, cooling, smoke detection, and other systems may not function properly and put people at risk. This is especially true for the oldest of elders because often their funds are limited, and maintaining or repairing a home is expensive.

Become a Sleuth

How can you tell when physical needs are becoming a problem? It is unusual for an elder to tap a loved one on the shoulder and say, "I'm having trouble moving around, driving, and preparing meals. Will you go to the doctor with me?" It happens, but rarely. It is more likely that a loved one will notice something that does not seem right. Family members often overlook or ignore the small changes in an elder, thinking, "That's just the way she is," or "He always…"

My dad grew up in rural Minnesota, and when he was in his forties, he told his father to go to Lake Itasca to see the Mississippi River's headwaters. Dad told my grandpa it was a beautiful place and you were not a Minnesotan without visiting there once. Everyone needs to step across the trickle of water that would grow into the mightiest river in the country. When my grandparents returned from their trip, Grandpa pulled Dad aside and berated him, saying, "We hated it up there! There were so many trees we couldn't see a thing!" He added a few expletives for emphasis. That conversation instantly entered our family's lore.

The cautionary tale is, "Don't miss the forest for the trees." That is the point when observing an elder. When we love and respect others we pay attention to them—who and how they are. Think of how a mother attends to the needs of her baby. She is kind, thoughtful, and nurturing—not missing a thing. That said, elders are not babies and should not be treated as such, but thoughtful attention and observation with which we honor them are vital. The key is paying attention, watching for clues that something might be going amiss.

Early detection and intervention of a potential problem is typically a good thing.

What kinds of things are important to observe? Many people are familiar with and can use Maslow's hierarchy of needs. The pyramid diagram shown below suggests that people strive to become their best selves but can advance only as each fundamental level's needs are met, starting from the base of the pyramid. So in theory, we likely do not focus on meeting our needs for esteem until our basic physiological, survival, and social needs are first met. There is some validity to the diagram, though scholars can debate elements of the examples listed.

Some elements are either unspoken or excluded from Maslow's hierarchy (which is why it is only a guide). That list might include spiritual needs (e.g., the need for salvation would likely be at the foundational level), and the need for each of us to contribute meaningfully to others is not clearly depicted in his pyramid. Regardless of possible shortcomings, consider using it as an observational tool. For example, start with observing the elder moving from the pyramid's base (primary human needs) and identify if the person's various needs are safely met at each level.

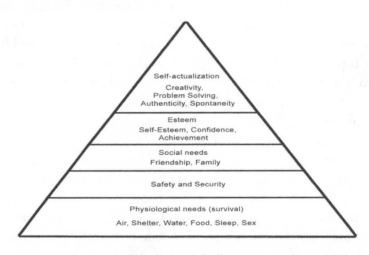

An alternative to using the pyramid is to consider the creation account in Genesis 1. God started with light, water, earth, and vegetation and separated day from night (creation days one through four, vv. 1–19). Each of these components of creation is essential to support life. Were any component absent, life as we know it could not occur. We can observe other ecosystems in the solar system that lack at least one essential component, and life cannot be sustained there.

On day five, God created the sea creatures, birds, and land animals (vv. 20–25) and called them "good" (v. 25). All of the higher creatures are sustained by the completeness (fulfillment) of the first four days of creation. On this fifth day, God prepared the purposes of humankind. These higher levels of life would help feed, clothe, and assist humans while providing them a reason (the need for purpose) for ruling over creation—the task given to them by God. On day six, God breathed into the dust and animated man, followed shortly by the woman (the need for family and companionship). Then he placed them into a garden (safety and security) to rule (esteem, divine purpose, achievement, and the activities of self-actualization).

While the illustration comparing Genesis 1 with Maslow's hierarchy is contrived and may be circular in reference, it is interesting to note how the Bible's first chapter reveals the order in which God's design meets our needs in a fashion predating Maslow's theory.

The actionable part of this analysis is if you cannot remember the order of Maslow's pyramid, think instead of the order of creation in Genesis 1 and see how each aspect is made (or not made) complete in the elder's life.

Genesis 1 and Maslow's hierarchy are convenient tools for providing observational cues, clues for watching anyone, including an elder. This is not advocating that people become judgmental; but that they become wise sleuths and intelligent in dialogue. When visiting the elder, casually look around, hold meaningful purpose-driven conversations. Consider bringing meals or snacks that require little preparation or cleaning up afterward. These "treats" create good reasons to look through cupboards and the refrigerator, make beverages, use the bathroom, etc. A note of caution, though: remember that we all have expired items in the bottom door of the fridge and the bathroom cabinet. A salad dressing bottle outdated by three years does necessarily indicate memory loss. Nor do cough drops that expired several months before. But it could show difficulty in bending down, reading small print, or distaste for cleaning the refrigerator and cabinets. The purpose is not to be the refrigerator police but to compassionately assist and retain the relationship while looking out for the person's best interest, as any caring friend would. Paul's exhortation in Romans 14:19 might apply here: "Let us therefore make every effort to do what leads to peace and mutual edification."

Below are some suggestions in what wise sleuths may look for:

- Physical environment: Observe their living quarters. Do they have heating and cooling and protection from the elements? Can they read the thermostat? Do the lights work, and are the lightbulbs in good condition? Do the utilities work? Do the ceilings show possible roof leaks? Is there a place for the elder to easily get up and down and rest? When were the smoke detector batteries last replaced? Does the elder have to climb stairs to the bedroom or bathroom, and are they safe doing so? Can they walk to and get up and down into chairs comfortably? Do they have a shower or a tub they can safely get into and out of? Is the home cluttered? Can they move a walker or cane throughout the house without catching on something? Are their scatter rugs? Are night-lights illuminating the way to the bathroom and kitchen? Does the plumbing or refrigerator icemaker leak?

  The operative action is to do everything necessary to eliminate potential slips, trips, or falls. Just assume the older person needs handrails in tubs and showers, around toilets and stairs, and help the elder select and install them. A quick internet search will turn up several attractive, non-institutional handrail and safety bar ideas. An older person may be upset to lose a favorite rug or to have furniture moved. But creating an open, uncluttered dry space with appropriate handholds is vital.

- Safety and security: Is the elder living in a place that is clean and has physical security (including freedom from abuse or neglect of any kind)? Are all areas free from trip and slip hazards? ("Make up your mind not to put any stumbling block or obstacle in your brother's way" [Rom. 14:13]). Gently inquire about how he gets food, medications, etc. Learn who and how often she sees her primary or other physicians and what medical issues the physicians are addressing. What kind of food is in the pantry or refrigerator, and is it safe (my mom had salad dressing in the refrigerator that was two years expired and a little sketchy lounging next to a variety of fresh vegetables)? The purpose is to ensure that the elder is safe and healthy.

- Social needs: Carry on a normal conversation. Inquire about who he sees and what kinds of social contacts he maintains. Find out how, and how often, she connects with others. Be a friend and learn about her friends, interests, and how she is retaining contact with a social network and community.

  Often elders of this generation have long connections to civic clubs, senior centers, or church groups. How are they interacting with multiple generations of people? Learn how they are keeping their world "large" and giving of themselves to others. Find out what they are learning or would like to learn. (As many people age, their world becomes smaller and smaller, which affects their sense of purpose and value. It may cause them to fear the outside world in an unhealthy way.)

- Esteem: As discussed earlier, we have been designed to live within family and community (think of family, clan, and tribe), and within that design are various roles and functions that help elders find and exercise purpose. Learn how the elder is doing that and what resources are being used so that he can contribute and continue to grow and experience life.

Make your visits pleasant, asking about the elder and his life. Having a meaningful conversation about day-to-day life can reveal many of the important things to know that will guide you in making necessary changes for the elder's health and safety. One aspect to

101

remember, though, is that it is a good idea to briefly write down your observations after a visit. They may become helpful should you have a growing concern and decide to accompany the elder on a visit with the primary care provider.

Outside of a disease process, the physical aspects that become problematic generally relate to not getting regular exercise and eating a healthy diet. This is because, over time, inadequate exercise and poor nutrition can decrease the ability to care for personal needs (dressing, toileting, and bathing). For example, many people's weight changes as they age. A significant weight loss may reduce an elder's muscle mass needed for adequate self-care. Too much weight gain can also hinder an elder's ability to exercise and care for personal needs. Thus, either too little or too much weight caused by inadequate exercise or inappropriate diet can limit an older person's ability to carry out the activities of daily living.

Through good observation and, as a compassionate friend, knowing what is happening in the elder's life gives clues to challenges that are not immediately obvious. It also may provide hints for simple things that can be done to interrupt a negative trend. Even modest strategies can address multiple levels of needs for a person. For example, taking an elder to church requires that he gets ready, gets into a vehicle, and walks into the building (physiological needs). There he may see family, friends, and acquaintances (social needs); worship God (spiritual needs—not depicted on Maslow's hierarchy); and be out of the home and seen and interact with others (which contribute to meeting the need for esteem).

Even if an elder is in assisted living or a nursing home, these seemingly simple experiences can provide great value on several levels for him or her. This is true even when memory loss is present. For example, there was an elder who lived with serious memory loss and spent an hour holding and playing with infants. Shortly after the children left, she remarked, "I don't know what I just did, but I sure feel good." Look for things the elders enjoy that will simultaneously meet multiple needs.

(The Resource section at the back of the book provides websites regarding observing elders.)

The Driving Need

Another contributor to physical decline is poor access to good nutrition and medicine. The financial relationship to this will be discussed later, but for now, an elder's loss of mobility can diminish his or her ability to remain independent. Mobility has multiple facets: retaining strength, balance, and flexibility to move around effectively, and the ability to prepare meals.

The further mobility issue is transportation: how does an elder physically get food and medicine? Numerous grocery stores, pharmacies, and runner services will deliver food and medicine. Friends or caregivers (family or paid) can also pick up food and other necessities. Many communities offer Meals on Wheels to elders. Most larger communities have taxi or bus services or elder transportation networks that help elders navigate independently as well. Many elders still have their cars and drive safely. In fact, many older drivers are the safest drivers on the road. However, we have all heard stories of elders who create driving hazards for the rest of us. An Insurance Institute for Highway Safety, Highway Loss Data Institute reports:

> Insurance claims provide another view of crashes of all severities. Drivers ages 65–69 have the lowest rates of property damage liability claims and collision claims per insured vehicle year. Rates start increasing after about age 70. However, older drivers' insurance claim rates are much lower than rates for the youngest drivers.[7]

It is a myth that all older drivers are bad drivers. However, driving can become more difficult for elders from a combination of diminishing eyesight, hearing loss, stiff joints, narrowing of peripheral clarity, slowing reflex times, physical limitations, and the stress they can cause.

Aging has a way of reducing peripheral vision both in how the eyes change and decreasing flexibility of the neck muscles and spine. As age progresses, the incidence of driver mishaps increases.

By retirement, most people have been driving for nearly half a century. Years of driving develop the driving process in a deep part of the brain, making driving something we can almost do unconsciously. Students and new drivers must engage higher levels of thought processes to drive. If they lose focus, they make mistakes, such as driving over curbs, missing stop signs, etc. But with some practice and hours behind the wheel, the same students become comfortable with driving and the mistakes decrease. This is all part of "learning" to drive. What is happening, though, is that many of the driving skills are being pushed deeper into the brain and becoming "automatic." Aging tends to slowly create barriers to the brain's access to those "automatic" skills through diminished sight, depth perception, peripheral vision, hearing, and reaction time. At times it appears that older drivers' skills move from being "automatic" to top of mind. The result may be slower speeds, enhanced caution, and anxious passengers.

Driving is considered a natural extension of our independent selves, and people often mistakenly perceive it as an inalienable right when, in truth, it is a privilege. When driving becomes unsafe for any reason, it is essential to address the cause or stop driving. Because people misperceive their aging abilities, that driving is a right and that decades of driving makes them safe, there is no easy way to remove a person's driving privileges. Generally, the depth of our attachment to driving is so deep, the loss of driving is tantamount to telling an elder, "You are no longer capable and independent." The loss of a vehicle and the ability to drive functionally limits the elder for transportation. Short of failing a required driving test (which is hard to fail) or having the license revoked due to an accident or other cause, few legal options are available—even when an elder may have serious memory loss.

While it is difficult to address driving issues with an elder, one of the less painful ways is to do so with other family members present and, possibly, the elder's doctor—and best done in a nonconfrontational manner and early (e.g., using a future tense "if this becomes the case") before any issues arise. It may be one of those conversations that occurs well before the elder has driving deficits. It can be an opportunity to educate what can often happen in older driver's health and experience that can make driving more difficult and riskier. Discuss alternatives to ensure the elder's transportation needs are met.

One family watched until their mother drove away from their home after a visit. As soon as she cleared the driveway, they called the police and reported a dangerous driver. The police pulled their mother over, gave her a ticket and a summons. She had to take another driver's test to get her license back. She passed the test and was back on the road. Finally, the family had to intervene. With the support of her doctor at a routine medical appointment, the family recommended she not drive due to her arthritis, poor hearing, and limited peripheral vision.

My mom drove her red Toyota Corolla to stores, restaurants, and church, often with friends on board. I noticed a bright yellow streak and dents down the passenger side of the car. When I asked her about her new "racing stripe," she said she had grazed a pillar in an underground garage. This was my opportunity to have "the talk" with her. Frankly, I chickened out. I missed a great chance to talk about narrowing peripheral vision and decreased vision from a poorly lit garage. I could have said, "The yellow stripe might be from the lighting and changes in vision. Let's get an eye appointment."

A better example is the daughters who spoke with their dad while he was in his mid-seventies. They said that it was not time for him to stop driving but asked when would he think it would be wise to give up the car. He was not willing to say, so they switched tactics and assured him that they were not recommending he give up driving then. But in the future, what might be the signals they all should watch for when the time was near? They agreed that should certain near misses, accidents, or health issues occur, it would be time to talk seriously about his no longer driving. They considered that there may come a time when he should limit his driving and what that might look like. They also discussed their chauffeuring him or finding transportation so he could continue to do the things he wanted to do. He did not like the conversation, but getting the topic out early and the caring family including him in the decision-making can work well.

One son went into his father's home and took his dad's keys. When Dad exploded at his son, the son said, "Dad, your driving is unsafe, and you're going to kill someone." This approach may cause long-lasting wounds and is normally recommended only as a last resort.

Driving is so much a part of some people's lives and self-image that one family left their dad's car in the parking lot of his assisted living building, even though the dad could no longer drive. He felt good that his car was there. He would occasionally get into the car and sit in the driver's seat.

One lady nearly lost her driver's license because she could not pass the eye exam. Her family consoled her and bought her a golf cart, which was slower; however, she was able to see and react properly while coasting along the retirement community sidewalk.

If the older person will listen to reason, it is best to have a team approach with the elder, sharing concerns about driving and what must happen. Demonstrating meaningful transportation alternatives ensures the elder still can live the life she or he has had (e.g., ways to get groceries, go to church or synagogue, meet with friends, eat out). Try not to have a family member become the "bully" in taking away keys. Instead, if there must be a bad guy, make it someone other than a family member or friend. Use an objective resource person (physician, social worker, law enforcement) so the family members can be supportive and helpful through a difficult situation. Family support will become essential if the elder experiences further losses in the time ahead. Do what you can to preserve healthy, positive family relationships; they will be needed for healthy support as the elder continues to age.

Being Thin-Skinned

One often-overlooked physical aspect bears discussion. Some elders' homes feel hot enough to sauté onions. Grandmas all over the country stop buying chocolates because they melt into amoebic masses in the cupboard. (Now you understand why there are chocolate chunks rather than chips in Grandma's cookies.) The high temperature is a common complaint of family and friends, accounts for large winter heating bills, and when mixed with the faint odor of mothballs, instantly transports many middle-aged people back to why visiting the great-grandparents was, well, "discomforting."

There is a physiological explanation for the high temperatures and the associated prohibition on open windows and fans. As we age, body composition changes. One of the changes is that the skin, the body's largest organ, tends to lose elasticity and thins (think wrinkles). This thinning contributes to heightened sensitivity to cool temperatures and breezes. So for many elders, a fan blowing directly at them is an uncomfortable physical sensation and makes them cold—doubly unpleasant. To be comfortable, the preference is to have room temperatures closer to the body core temperature (98.6 Fahrenheit). Okay, it may not really be 98.6 in Grandma's house, but it is common to keep the room at a higher temperature and draft-free. One way to address the warmth issue is to keep sweaters or shawls around the house for elders when they visit, recognizing that the elder needs warmer temperatures to feel comfortable. Remember, the elder's home may be warmer for their comfort, so when visiting, dress in layers that can be removed as needed.

As the skin thins, it creates the potential for other issues compounded by the need for warmth. First, because of the thinning skin, elders are naturally more susceptible to hypothermia and dehydration. Fluctuations of temperature, and low temperatures, can have serious consequences for elders. Second, when the body is warm, the skin pores open, allowing water and chemicals to pass through the skin more easily. The greatest concern with high room temperature is that it is dehydrating. Dehydration can cause or contribute to several issues, including hospitalization and death. It can also be exacerbated by disease (e.g., diabetes), poor nutrition, medications, alcohol, sweating, kidney problems, and more. Dehydration can also contribute to diabetic issues and bladder infections, which can increase the effect of other issues.

Some articles suggest that elders often forget to drink because they may not feel thirsty. Or when they drink more, they need to use the bathroom more, creating more issues if the person is incontinent. For some people, mobility limitations are worse to deal with than thirst. Still, it is important to ensure that elders drink enough fluids. Be sure to discuss dehydration risk with the elder and his or her primary care provider for recommendations to help avoid problems.

As simple as the solution is, dehydration alone can cause an emergency room visit. Clues to look for include dry lips or mouth, fatigue, concentrated urine, and lightheadedness. New fluids are available that reportedly reduce dehydration and the loss of vital nutrients without requiring more bathroom stops. If they are affordable for the elder, they may be a good alternative.

Changes in How Food Tastes

My brother and I loved our German grandmother dearly but hated eating at her house. She was a delightful lady, but we swore everything she prepared was pickled and overcooked, including fish and beets. It all tasted and smelled like vinegar. Mom told us that when Grandma was a farm mother of seven, vinegar was an affordable preservative. Meat was not inspected, as it is today, and had to be cooked well done for safety. Being a good mom, she always cooked things thoroughly and pickled stuff liberally. As she aged, it seemed as if she was using an increasing amount of vinegar. In retrospect, I do not know if that was due to a loss of or decrease in taste, physical decline, or simply the lifelong practice of using a strong flavor. Maybe it is what she liked best, and she shared it with us.

Compelled to Be Proactive?

Why should we look for and address gradual physical changes as well as health and safety with an elder? The earlier discussion supplied insight, though a few more facts underscore why it is important not to ignore subtle or significant changes you may see in the elder(s) in your life.

As we learned earlier, the risks of dying within a year following major surgery increases with age. In a Finnish study, the authors concluded that "During the study period, the risk of mortality in hip fracture patients was 3-fold higher than that in the general population and included every major cause of death."[8]

They also found that approximately 79 percent of people over the age of eighty-five died within a year of surgery to repair a fractured hip.[9] More studies report similar outcomes with other major surgery on elders over eighty-five. An elder in a nursing home has a higher risk of dying from invasive surgery than those of the same age living at home. Of course, a person in a nursing home may have more comorbidities or higher frailty. "Even when the researchers matched these two groups of patients by age and by the number of other diseases they had, those in the nursing home group (and in this study that meant long-term residents, not those in temporary rehab) were significantly more likely to die in each case."[10] The study does not explain the difference in mortality between people in nursing homes and those going home. It is not necessarily an indictment of nursing homes as much as it underscores a person at home may perform more activities of daily living and exercise to retain independence. It is a question worth more study. Two points we should take away from this. First, as the above quote points out, a key question to ask before the surgeon scrubs is if there are any alternatives to surgery to try first. This is particularly true for the older person frail enough to require nursing home care. Second, safety does matter to elders. Prevention of falls and accidents is paramount to saving lives.

Application

The elder's physician is a key ally in helping an elder to be safe and healthy. People do not always remember everything from discussions with health-care providers, so it is helpful for an appropriate family member to accompany the elder to physician visits and take notes. Issues and concerns can be brought out in discussion in ways that the elder leads the conversation (or at least is a willing participant) with the physician. The idea is that, presuming the elder is loved and respected, helpers will retain a supportive perspective in the elder maintaining control.

If issues are to be confronted, enlist the support of the health-care professionals who have a trusted, positive, objective relationship with the elder. Keep in mind that as adults, elders have the right to refuse whatever they do not want. Their choices are their responsibility unless they have been legally adjudicated incompetent by a court. At times, the aged will make decisions that may not seem wise to us. That is particularly difficult when the person we love or feel responsible for makes decisions we believe are ill considered or unwise.

Without giving names, think briefly about a visit you recently had in a friend's or elder's home. What do you remember observing?

Talk about the steps you might take to observe a loved one's home life.

Think about doing the observations discussed in this chapter. How would you feel if a friend observed you in your home? What if you did not know they were making the observations but told you later? How would you feel?

Takeaway Thoughts

People do not suddenly transform from midlife to old. Instead, the process of aging is a continuous transition in which the whole of who we become is greater than the sum of all our experiences.

We change as we age, and how we are in our older years is at least in part determined by our meals (nutrition), medications (health care), exercise, and social connectedness.

The sheer number of people turning sixty-five today is greater than any previous generation. With lower birth rates, the number of people in retirement will proportionately be large enough to redirect some aspects of our culture and how the government sets priorities through legislation and allocates tax dollars.

It is not unusual for a ninety-year-old person to have children entering retirement. Determining what the older people in our lives need to maximize their independence takes careful watching and listening—a little bit of detective work.

Transportation can be a challenging issue for older people. Living in a walkable community or a place where golf carts are welcomed can be helpful, but this is not an option for many people. Driving is one of the last bastions of independence and can be necessary to obtain food, medications, and other things. After driving for sixty or seventy years, it is extremely difficult to give up and produces challenges and dangers all their own.

Skin becomes thinner as we age. It means that older people may feel colder and be sensitive to fans or moving air and explains why they often keep the thermostat on warmer settings. Their thinner skin makes them more subject to dehydration, which occurs faster in warmer rooms.

Falls among the aging are particularly dangerous and can result in premature mortality. Taking action to prevent falls is paramount to helping elders retain their best quality of life.

The risk of major surgery increases with age. Avoiding surgery has two aspects. The first is staying safe, particularly from trip hazards and falling. The second is that less invasive forms of treatment should be seriously considered for people in their eighties (or younger in the presence of comorbidities) and beyond if options available.

Questions for Consideration

1. From chapter 1 we learned that we were designed to age. Our experience is that we transition through our entire lives. What do you think the benefits of constant transition are once we reach the age of fifty, seventy-five, or ninety?
2. How much of our physical changes do you think are due to the great corruption versus lifestyle choices?
3. How do you morally and ethically observe another person's life and then make decisions to act on his or her benefit?
4. Using what you know about God's design and purpose for us and the protection of family and community, how might you discuss your observations with the elder in your life?

5. How might fear of safety or loss of independence affect the above conversation? Could those fears impel healthy changes of behavior? How?

6. Have you ever been in an elder's home or room and felt the temperature was too high? What did you do/say?

6

Property, Money, and Aging

You can be young without money, but you can't be old without it.
—Tennessee Williams
(*Cat on a Hot Tin Roof*)

Money provides choices and options. As a person's money increases, so do their choices and options. Recent research suggests that the richest people live the longest. Money, by itself, does not add years to life or life to years, but it is a resource to enhance their health, nutrition, and exercise. Like so many things, the secret is how we use resources for the greatest benefit.

Use of Resources

In the 1970s, a ninety-year-old woman lived near a small village in the Bavarian mountains. She lived alone, was not well to do, and her home was small with a tiny kitchen and few cupboards. Six days a week, rain or shine, she walked over a mile up a high, steep mountain path to go to market. At the market, she chatted with the farmers and friends for an hour or so and sometimes shared a cup of thick dark coffee with a friend. She returned home with her few purchases and made a simple dinner. On Sundays, there was no market, but she walked up to the village to attend church and visit with friends and relatives.

She befriended some American students studying in the town who occasionally offered to drive her home. Unless the weather was bad, she refused the ride, saying the walk kept her strong. One day some of the students visited her home and offered to hike up the mountain with her. As they climbed the hill in the thin mountain air, the students could not keep conversing with her because the climb was so difficult. They were amazed she could make the climb every day.

While the woman had little money and her options were limited, she used her few resources very well. She created a healthy lifestyle through simple, inexpensive choices. The daily climb was great exercise, and carrying the groceries down the hill was her weight training. Maintaining significant social contacts combined with simple nutrition provided significant positive health benefits. The deciding factor in how she used her resources was her attitude—she decided that she was responsible for her choices and that she would be a blessing to others, not a burden. She excelled at living because she decided that funds did not limit her. They were enough regardless of their face value.

Doris moved into a retirement village in the late 1970s that later went bankrupt. The organization had promised her "life care," meaning that once she put up a large entry fee, her monthly cost there would remain relatively flat, even if she lived in the most expensive area. The financial failure of the organization left her vulnerable to the new nonprofit corporation that rescued the business. Due to the bankruptcy, she did not have enough money to either underwrite a new life-care contract or move out. If Doris eventually moved to the nursing home, she would have to pay a higher rate, and she would run out of money.

The new company obtained a Medicaid agreement with the state and promised not to move anyone out because of the inability to pay. These assurances helped the lady greatly. However, she said, "I gave the bulk of my assets to the first organization in the original entry fee. I have just enough to live on now, but it is too little for me to move. I no longer have a choice. The new company assures me that I will be cared for, but I feel so vulnerable. You see, I am in my early eighties and have no chance to recoup my losses." (Please note the failure of retirement communities though rare, does occasionally occur. The new owner was a well-run, nonprofit organization that recreated the community in which the residents were able to thrive securely and happily for the balance of their lives.) The point is, financially, elders have little time to recover from a major expense or loss. Often, few people can help Doris and those like her whose funds are depleted through no fault of their own.

God's design in the law was unique in how it required family support, property valuation, interest-free loans, and the return of assets during the Jubilee year. Centuries before the concept of government assistance, the law essentially guaranteed the provision for every elder, infirm, and poor person. Paul speaks of that responsibility in the New Testament book of 1 Timothy (more on that later).

Today, it is common for an elder to live thirty or even forty years after retiring. Many people's retirement funds do not last, or they diminish from inflation, economic woes, or unexpected medical costs. What was once considered "enough" retirement funds may no longer be. Sadly, as older people experience some of these financial issues, they tap into their assets. But their income decreases because they have fewer assets to invest. A spiral begins: as they draw down the assets to live on, their income drops until they eliminate their assets and much of their income. Those relying on US Social Security benefits find that the cost of living rises faster than their monthly payments. Unfortunately, as people approach the outward limit of their physical bodies, the cost of medical interventions tends to increase. Even with various programs, insurances, and Medicare, physician visits, lab tests and imaging, medical procedures, drugs, other therapies, etc., are expensive. Paying for health care and diagnostics can rapidly deplete the financial reserves of elders. It is not uncommon for the exhaustion of funds to occur with one elder while the spouse may have years of living ahead with lower income, heavy medical and funeral bills, and greatly diminished assets.

Being good stewards of our physical health affects us most in the later years of life. The financial impact of our physical stewardship likely lowers demands for health care, particularly as we age past eighty or eighty-five. The data from the baby boomer generation is not yet in, but anecdotally this stands to reason.

How Much Money Is Enough?

How much is enough? Should our goal be to
    have money left when we die? The psalmist
    wrote:
Do not be overawed when a man grows rich,
when the splendor of his house increases;
for he will take nothing with him when he dies,
his splendor will not descend with him.
Though while he lived he counted himself
    blessed—
and men praise you when you prosper. (Ps.
    49:16–20)

Do not wear yourself out to get rich;
have the wisdom to show restraint.
Cast but a glance at riches and they are gone,
For they will surely sprout wings and fly off to
    the sky like an eagle. (Prov. 23:4–5)

The Scriptures, as well as life, teach that not everyone will be wealthy in this life. It is prudent to save and set aside funds for the future as each person is blessed. God's design in supporting the aging and the poor indicates his concern for people in need. He wants us to have a similar perspective. In the Jewish law, God set a structure to transfer wealth and property so elders would have advocates, responsible caregivers, and the funds to ensure their lifelong care. Inheritance was not just about money and valuables; it was a transfer of family responsibility.

The healthiest attitude about an elder's money is for the family to encourage the elder to use the funds as the older person deems wise. She earned it, and it is hers to use and enjoy, whether it is giving a substantial amount away, going on trips, or setting up the grandchildren's college funds. If an elder has memory or other mental issues, it may be wise to modify this to include an objective person to help maximize the elder's quality of life while not risking foolish spending or getting scammed.

Issues arise rapidly when heirs create expectations, thinking they "deserve" an inheritance, or they begin prespending an elder relative's money. The mature, ethical perspective is to realize that the money an elder earned or has is for the elder's benefit. Having money left after death is fine, but focusing on the elder's well-being and life enjoyment is the best for sleeping soundly at night.

The tax codes set legal limits to giving away money. Please note that should the elder ever need public assistance, many governmental entities require a five-year or longer "look back" into an elder's financial records for gifts given to family, misspent or hidden assets, etc. If substantial gifts are given away, the elder may be disqualified from receiving public assistance until those funds are repaid for the elder's benefit. (As a rule, it is wise to obtain legal and tax advice before giving substantial sums of money to anyone.) It is also wise to ensure that good records of the elder's use of their funds are maintained. At some point, and for a variety of reasons, good records could become vital.

Keeping Assets in the Family Is a Good Thing, Right?

"The greedy stir up conflict, but those who trust in the LORD will prosper" (Prov. 28:25).

Chapter 2 described how, in ancient Israel, property was to revert to the original family ownership at the time of the Jubilee. However, shrewd businessmen and lawyers found a way within the law to retain possession. They declared the land as Corban, "a gift to the Lord." Technically, then, the property was given to the Lord. Using this tactic, the land would not revert to the original family, while making the shrewd person appear righteous and God honoring (to those who did not know the truth). And the one declaring the land Corban would retain the right to work the land. This is essentially the same justification of a youngster who palms the money he is supposed to put in the offering plate at church. In either case, the perpetrator is saying, "I'll look like I'm doing something good, but really, God wants me to have this," or "I am more deserving of this because…" or "This is going to be shared anyway. I'll just cut out the middleman."

With a Corban gift, technically the Lord owned the property, and the property managers were just tenants and remained so in perpetuity. The payment to the Lord for use of the property was 10 percent of the crops or the crop value. In this practice, the shrewd person would keep control of the property, take 90 percent of the profits. The crafty tenant looked "righteous" but did not pay rent for the property, did not have the family responsibilities associated with the property, and had a greater profit. There was little downside to this cunning person. Jesus repudiated this kind of practice:

> And [Jesus] said to [the Pharisees and teach-
> ers of the law]: "You have a fine way of setting
> aside the commands of God to observe your own
> traditions! For Moses said, 'Honor your father and
> your mother,' and 'Anyone who curses his father
> or mother must be put to death.' But you say that
> if a man says to his father or mother: 'Whatever
> help you might otherwise have received from me
> is Corban' (that is, a gift devoted to God), then
> you no longer let him do anything for his father
> or mother. Thus, you nullify the word of God by
> your tradition that you have handed down. And
> you do many things like that." (Mark 7:9–13)

A similar scheme might be played today in which an elder retitles his house or other assets in an adult child's name for a dollar; then years later (when there is a financial need or government assistance requirement), the elder technically has no assets. Unfortunately, there are times when the adult child, who now has the house and assets, takes little or no responsibility for the elder's needs. This transfer of assets may be done with good intentions but can be viewed as an attempt to pass the responsibility of care and services from the elder and family to the public trust. It may also create an elder's expectation that a family member will take care of him but does not materialize. In this case, the elder may feel simultaneously swindled and neglected. Hard feelings can echo through the family for years.

God's plan is for us to care for the aged and poor. While social structures are in place to help ensure elders receive the services they need, it remains implicit in the passage above that we have a responsibility to do both what we can and what is right. We are not responsible for what we cannot do, for that is inconsistent with God's justice and compassion. But we are to do what we can.

Some people take their elders' assets and by legal means set the money into protected accounts so that if Mom or Dad go into the nursing home, they will quickly qualify for public assistance. This method "shields" the elders' funds from use in their care while employing public tax dollars to pay for their services. That way the heirs receive far more assets, and the parents still get care. This tactic ignores that the elder's family is first responsible for the care of the elder (one responsibility of inheritance). While they may have met the moral responsibility (Mom is still getting the care, regardless of payer source, says the law), they are crossing an ethical boundary by using public tax dollars to care for someone who has sufficient funds.

Another concern is that in long-term care, public assistance does not pay the full cost of care for individuals, and about 66 percent of people in nursing homes are on public assistance. To make up for the incomplete payment for people on public assistance, private pay and insurance clients must pay more to provide care. Government sources argue that they pay the "full cost of care" for people on public assistance. The problem is that the government determines what the full cost of care means, and long-term care businesses usually cannot survive only on what the government defines as allowable—*allowed* and *appropriate* are two entirely different matters.

Government programs like Medicaid are among the greatest annual budget items the states have. With benefits codified in state and federal laws, the states have little latitude in controlling the cost of that budget item. According to one source, Medicaid alone accounted for an average of 29 percent of total state budget dollars in fiscal year 2018.[1]

Again, we must ask: How much money is enough as we age? We all want to live well and to remain independent for life, without having to turn to family, friends, or the government for support. Each of our circumstances is unique. Compare what you reasonably think your expenses will be with your sources of income. A trustworthy financial planner can help make estimates of future needs. Remember, though, your future is in God's hands, and you could have significant health-care expenses in the later years of life…or not.

If your expenses are greater than your income, you have three choices: (1) increase income, (2) decrease expenses, or (3) figure out what assistance is available. None of us knows the future; it is in God's hands. We are to be prudent and wise, knowing that, like the old woman who lived near the mountain village, the objective is to use our resources wisely to sustain meaningful purpose in a God-honoring life. While money helps make that appear easier to accomplish, it is far from the only thing. As Paul wrote in Philippians 1:21–22, "For to me, to live is Christ and to die is gain. If I am to go on living in the body, this will mean fruitful labor for me." The reality is that at times, some of the most influential people in our communities are elders who have little money but give much in life.

Retirement Communities

Ask a few friends what a retirement community is; then ask them to define a Life Plan Community. Finally, ask them how a Life Plan Community, by their definition, is different from assisted living, congregate care, catered living, and a nursing home. You get the picture. These names are nice terms for nursing homes, right? If you agree to that statement, then you might also agree that all cars are just differently named Fords. There is a substantive difference between all car manufacturers just as there are vast differences in the terms used to describe long-term care options.

There are distinctly different care locations, whose definitions can differ between states. The differences in these terms are available on the internet (AARP has some particularly good information, as do many sites serving senior adults). Let us take a look at a brief list of terms.

Nursing Home

A nursing home is an institution serving four or more unrelated people and is licensed by the state to provide twenty-four-hour care and services supervised by licensed nurses and other personnel. The plan of care is based on an assessment of the individual. A physician must assess the person and state that the elder requires nursing home care. The nursing home is responsible for providing all necessary care and services (though not for the payment of all services). The elders living in nursing homes generally stay in rooms (as opposed to apartments), and many share the room with another unrelated elder. Most nursing homes contract with the federal government to provide Medicare (insurance) services. Most nursing homes also contract with the state to provide care for elders needing public assistance (called Medicaid in most states).

Assisted Living

Assisted living is an institution serving four or more unrelated people, licensed by the state to provide a living environment with the level of services provided as individually contracted with each person living there. While many assisted living facilities' apartments have small kitchenettes, three meals a day are normally provided in the main dining area, like a hotel dining room. Assisted living licenses allow them to provide elders with hands-on care for personal needs, as well as medication assistance supervised by a nurse. Upon entry, the individual and the institution enact a service plan. If a person living there needs twenty-four-hour supervision over a certain number of days, the state regulations (which differ by state) may require them to move into a nursing home or other supervised environment. Generally, assisted living is paid from the personal funds of the elders or their families. Some states do have public assistance programs for assisted living services.

Congregate Living

Like assisted living, congregate living provides contracted services to each individual but typically provides less intense hands-on care than assisted living (depending on the state). Usually, the living setting is an apartment building with some meal services available each day. Housekeeping and other services are available as part of the monthly fee, with an additional menu of services available. In some states, assisted living centers may be called congregate living.

Catered Living

Often, catered living is a type of congregate living but with most services based on a menu of prices rather than being all-inclusive. Think of this in terms of living in a suite hotel with a variety of available services; only it is set up to help the elder remain independent.

Independent Living

This is what it sounds like: patio homes or apartment-style living for elders who can live independently (which has a variety of definitions). While several different types of contracts differentiate between the pricing and structure of services, these typically are paid for through either an entry fee arrangement with a monthly fee or a monthly rental. They are often on a campus that provides several features and amenities, including optional dining services, emergency staff, maintenance, grounds keeping, and housekeeping.

Life Plan Community or Continuing Care Retirement Communities (CCRC)

These organizations offer multiple levels of the above services in a campus arrangement. They usually provide independent living and various levels of assisted living and nursing home services. Many offer a panoply of additional features such as wellness life-styles, fitness areas with pools, multiple public and dining venues, and planned events. The larger CCRCs often have arrangements for home health, clinics, and a multitude of services. The variety and strength of services available are based on the concept that elders will move through a continuum of services where they remain in one community surrounded by people they know and are close to friends. This concept provides security for individuals who know up front where they can get assistance as needed. Anecdotal research suggests that elders who choose to move into Life Plan Communities may have up to four or more years of quality independent living than those who remain in their homes. The reasons for this extension of quality days are not well understood, though it is believed to be either from the robust sense of living many people have from being in a community environment with supportive services easily accessible. Others suggest that elders who move into CCRCs may just be healthier due to their prior life choices.

Life Care

This type of Life Plan Community contracts with elders to provide care and services for the balance of their lives at a predetermined monthly fee, regardless of where they live on campus.

Because states and providers use different names for the various levels of care, it can best be known what a provider offers by asking them. As someone once said, "If you've been to one Life Plan Community, you've been to only one Life Plan Community." They offer similar services under different names and in different ways.

The way Life Plan Communities operate is evolving as health alternatives and funding becomes available. People, who once would have been found only in nursing homes, may remain in their apartments with medication supervision and personal assistance. Someone requiring assistance with their activities of daily living (bathing, dressing, eating, etc.) may live in assisted living though they technically could qualify for nursing home care. The evolution in caregiving is that rather than moving people from one level to another to receive more care, the care is brought to the person in their choice of environments (if they can afford it).

Long-Term Care Insurance

How does long-term care insurance play into an elder's planning? A variety of plans and programs are available, but, generally, for each day a person receives eligible long-term care services, the insurance company pays a predefined benefit. Two things should be kept in mind. The first is that long-term care insurance is a program that protects the elder's funds. It can be expensive insurance, and if the elder does not have many assets (i.e., they will likely be on public assistance within a year or two of entering long-term care), it may not be worth the cost. Like anything, though, a person who has more money has more choices, and the insurance may help provide options as to where care is received while helping to protect assets. Be cautious, however, because if the elder does not have many assets, a long-term care policy might disqualify her from public assistance and receiving needed care. As stated in Proverbs, "In the multitude of counselors there is wisdom." Get good advice from reliable sources.

The second consideration is what does *long-term care service* mean? Insurance companies define long-term care differently. This key definition is sometimes buried in the fine print. It is not uncommon for insurance agents selling long-term care products to be unfamiliar with the full spectrum of possible long-term care services—and some locations of the country do not have a lot of options. The policy documents specifically define what services are paid for, which are not, and what criteria must be met prior to qualifying for payment. For example, an elder may have had surgery and need someone to come to their home five days a week for homemaking services: cooking, cleaning, and laundry. They may receive this service through a home health or private-duty or personal care service. Frankly, many maid services could do the same things in an elder's home. The question is, will the insurance cover any of the services? Some do if the service is ordered by a physician and provided by a licensed home health or home care agency. Other policies will not pay for this service. It varies by company and policy.

To answer the question of qualifying for payment, think about the likely scenarios the elder may experience. If no other caregivers are in the home or the area, a more robust policy might be advisable. If the elder has a lot of family and community support, a different policy may be more cost-effective. The key is to plan what you think are likely scenarios. The elder's primary care provider, hospital discharge planners, or senior citizen center social workers can provide good insight into what elders do for care in the area when needed. Through this planning, a wise family member can often preplan options for care with the elder using the phrase, "Should you ever need…" or my favorite, the less frightening airline disclaimer, "In the unlikely event of…"

Long-term care itself is complicated. It may be unreasonable to expect that all people who sell long-term care insurance know all of the nuances of the field, though they should know their policies well. If you are interested in long-term care insurance, it may be wise to run the policy past someone with administrative or executive experience or knowledge of long-term care. Many state consumer advocates or insurance regulation offices may be helpful in this area too.

Today, fewer people are receiving retirement money through defined pension plans, and a significant number of people have retirement annuities. Regarding pensions (and sometimes annuities) at retirement, the recipient selects whether the benefit amount is to be paid on their lifetime only or whichever spouse lives the longest (or the shortest!). It is easy to look at the difference in the monthly amount to be received and select the higher payment. After all, two people need more to live on than one, right? The problem is that often the person receiving the pension or annuity (frequently the male) dies before the spouse, leaving the surviving spouse without the pension. Many times I have had to walk on eggshells around widows whose incomes largely passed away with their husbands. In the difficult financial moments, they are not fondly remembering the person who was hailed as their protector. No one knows which spouse will die first, though statistically males often go before their female spouses. So be aware of how the loss of one spouse's income will affect the bereaved.

Someone once said that the only sure things in life are birth, death, and taxes, and with death, there are still taxes. Many people do not think about the reportable income the year they die. So we pay taxes after we are dead, at least our estates do for us. One fellow reportedly told the IRS that when he goes to the grave, his final tax check will be in his pocket, but they will need to come and get it. The story may be an urban legend, but the truth is that the estate pays the taxes. That means when we die, someone must sort through our papers and stuff to complete the estate. In short, a family member once said that he thought his mother loved him until she named him executor.

It is important to have both a will and a living will. But that is not enough. It helps to preplan the burial fees and funeral arrangements as well. But that still is not enough. Get your financial papers in order, name the executor early, and provide them everything they need for an orderly transition. Even people with few funds can unintentionally make things extremely difficult for an executor by lack of documentation, disorganized records, and multiple diversifications of assets. Have the information easily accessible for the executor. Perhaps file it with an attorney or other safe place, and have it summarized and ready to go when you pass. These things are also important should an elder need public assistance of any kind, because the various governmental programs will require the verification of all funds before any public benefit is allowed.

Unethical Financial Solicitors

The ninety-three-year-old woman walked into my office one day, immediately followed by a sheriff's detective. I could tell she had been crying and still had spasms of inconsolable crying. I immediately turned to her and said her name, but she would not look up at me. I offered her a box of tissues and said, "I know there is deep loss here, please help me understand."

The detective spoke quietly. "Anna has had most of her money stolen by scammers from outside the country. The callers said they were part of a Christian mission and had befriended her. They kept calling her back with updates, telling her of greater needs and requests until they nearly cleared out her bank account."

Anna, filled with emotion, declared, "I am such an idiot! It was my fault! I gave all my money away to scammers." Sobbing, she could not speak for a while.

We reminded her that she was secure living in our organization and that scammers are professionals who prey on people. As professionals they sound legitimate, smooth, and truthful; in reality, they are professional liars and swindlers. She was victimized just as if they had broken into her home and stolen her money. She was close to her pastor who, with us and the detective, helped her obtain counseling and other services.

In the following weeks, we invited the detective to speak to groups of older people living in our senior community about how elders are often targeted by scammers, how to detect and avoid them, and what to do should they get scammed. (Of course, Anna's name was not used and is not her real name in any case.)

Later, when the detective and I were visiting one afternoon, he commented that most elders do not report scamming to the police because they are ashamed for falling for the ruse. They feel so stupid that they do not want anyone to know. They recognize they are victims and are ashamed that they allowed themselves to be victimized. The detective's full-time job was following up with people who had been scammed. He said it is often difficult to charge and prosecute the scammers because many times they live and work from one of several foreign countries. US law has no jurisdiction outside its borders, and various treaties and relationships are not in place for police to pursue those criminals.

But people in this country, including friends and family, occasionally scam elder funds. One way to avoid this is to have several trusted people with access to view the information in an elder's various funds. They can observe how funds are being spent while not necessarily having access to the money. If unexplained irregularities are found in a senior's spending, it is wise to consider it carefully, possibly involve a lawyer or adult protective services, and notify law enforcement as needed.

Some families have joint accounts with the elder. Usually, it is a POA who keeps an eye out for unusual expenses to help protect the elder. Some accounts can require two signatures for checks or withdrawals over a certain amount to reduce the likelihood of a stolen checkbook in which someone tries to drain an account. Other families have the mail sent to their homes first and then deliver it to the elder. This helps prevent someone outside the family from getting account numbers and statements by stealing mail.

Finances and End-of-Life Care

Few issues garner attention and emotion as the discussion of finances and end-of-life care. The changes in American health-care law and practice will force this sensitive issue into a national dialogue at some point. In this section we will look at some of the reasons why a societal dialogue is needed and underscore a moral and scriptural perspective on this very divisive topic. This discussion here is from a distinctly biblical perspective: Scripture teaches there is dignity, purpose, and sanctity to life. God's original design was not influenced by death until the "great corruption" (see chapter 1). While we were intended to age, death does not bring God any pleasure (Ezek. 18:32). Research may help illustrate an answer that honors the scriptural perspective and creates helpful dialogue in managing scarce personal and societal funds. Frankly, though, the facts in this section take the reader into difficult ethical and moral territory, which is why the starting point is based on the Scripture's teaching of the sanctity of life.

End-of-life care will at some point enter the national debate. It is estimated that about 5 percent of people receiving Medicare use a range of between 13 and 21 percent of the Medicare dollars spent each year (depending on the model assumptions). This 5 percent are the Medicare recipients who are in the last twelve months of their lives.

> The percentage of Medicare's cost represented by 2015 decedents rises to 21%. This percentage is somewhat lower than that reported by Riley and Lubitz based upon Medicare data between 1978 and 2006, although these authors report a decreasing trend in EOL costs. The percentage is higher than that reported by other authors, likely because we include a full 12 months of final year expenses for decedents and defer the current year's final 12-month costs for those members who die in the following year.[2]

The costs increase exponentially by the location in which care is received with inpatient hospital costs exceeding hospice or nursing home care by a factor of five to ten.

> Average Medicare expenditures per decedent per month are greater in the last 90 days preceding death versus the last 180 days preceding death, confirming the exponential increase in costs as death approaches. The highest spending occurs in acute hospitals. Care provided in skilled nursing, hospice, and home health care are other major sources of Medicare expenditures.[3]

This expenditure raises moral and ethical dilemmas ranging from the sanctity of life discussion to questioning why 5 percent of people should receive up to 25 percent of the money while leaving 95 percent of recipients to share the balance? Should or can the funds somehow be reallocated for greater social good? And who should be the decision makers and control the funds: physicians, families, patients, or bankers and bureaucrats? When the Affordable Care Act was being debated, just the whisper of limiting funds for people in the last year of life suddenly became a discussion of "death squads" and other such terms. Inflammatory language aside, what are the facts? Death is unpredictable. Nearly a quarter of Medicare dollars are spent on 5 percent of Medicare recipients whose mortality is above 50 percent in their last year of life. The other 95 percent is used for people who have a lower likelihood of dying but in the end, do.[4]

The psalmist wrote, "I am fearfully and wonderfully made." Life and health are not entirely predictable. When statisticians review Medicare, they see that about 21 percent of the spending is during the last twelve months of life. As people near death, the cost of care increases exponentially. However, when tracking the Medicare dollars used by people medical professionals presume will die in a year with a probability of dying greater than 50 percent, the spending drops to 13 percent.

What does this mean? First, medicine is both art and science. Practitioners cannot predict a disparate group of people's ends of life—who will live and who will die. They can offer percentages and likelihoods, but as the Teacher says, "As no one has power over the wind to contain it, no one has the power over the time of their death" (Eccles. 8:8).

Second, since the exact timing of a person's end of life due to diminishing health is not predictable, how can people know whether they should undergo aggressive treatment or not? The US health-care system is designed for individuals, with the advice of professionals who are not all knowing, to make their choices for care. That decision is based on the experience of practitioners and the patient's perspective, knowledge, faith, and human and financial resources.

Third, it is common for families to make emotional decisions relating to end-of-life care. Anecdotally, many families send a beloved parent to the hospital from home or the nursing home to have the parent subsequently pass away at the hospital within hours or days. Despite the opinions or advice of their physicians and other professionals, many times families send their loved ones to the hospital when little can be done for them. The question to be asked here is not financial. Instead, it is an emotional decision: Is the hospital the best place to die? Hospitals are good places for healing but they are unable to have the knowledge and relationship with an elder due to their short time together. Often an elder living at a nursing home or assisted living knows the staff well and may be more comfortable dying with people around them they know and care about. Likewise, the staff work hard to ensure a safe and dignified passing for an elder they know and care about. It would serve families well to discuss with their loved ones prior to such an event what the elder desires and what is the best for him or her.

The discussion of how the allocation of elder health-care dollars and end-of-life decisions should be made will likely be fronted with limited financial resources considering the best use of those resources. Should an informed individual be able to make a decision that costs society significant resources without that same society having a voice? The devil's advocate could suggest that those end-of-life resources might be better spent in ways to improve other people's health that will bring about greater social good. For example, if the poor had better and more access to health care, and the dollars were spent to improve their social determinants of health (housing, nutrition, etc.), the social benefit could be huge in terms of lives saved, length of life improved, and the social and financial (tax dollars) return of that group. Preventive care in this scenario could have an enormous return to society.

The social good argument is powerful. Yet at the basis of the perspective is that the Scriptures tell us that *all* life is valuable and is to be valued. Is the social argument ultimately based on the cultural assumption that younger people are more valuable than elders? What if we were to value elders more than we do now and learn to both enhance and expand their influence and knowledge? Could that also have a significant societal impact? Ascribing value, importance, and purpose to older people could have a profound impact on our culture, increasing life satisfaction to the degree that their health-care costs might decline. How is this possible? A person with hope and a purpose is more likely to take care of themselves throughout life. If "retirement" were to become a retirement *to* something rather than a retirement *from* a valued state, younger people would likely care better for themselves, reducing social costs across their entire lifespans.

Older people use the highest percentage of health-care costs. This is in no way to imply that we should seek to hasten death or withhold care. However, this does make the argument for finding different methods of allocating the health-care dollar. David wrote in Psalm 6:4–5, "Turn, O LORD, and deliver me; save me because of your unfailing love. No one remembers you when you are dead. Who praises you from the grave?" And "I take no pleasure in the death of anyone, declares the Sovereign LORD" (Ezek. 18:32).

What is the answer regarding end-of-life care and the distribution of the dollars for that care? Since God designed and created us and has great compassion for us, it is clear the sanctity of life is inviolate. If moral principle, choice, and the drive to sustain self all embrace the "do everything you can for as long as you can" mode of thinking, is that necessarily the best alternative for the individual, the surviving spouse and loved ones, and society at large? It makes sense that this perspective is predominant regarding end-of-life care and its financial and social cost—people want to remain alive and in the best ability their conditions allow for as long as possible.

Part of the answer may be found in the literature regarding the use of hospice care. While more research needs to be done, *Reuters Health* reported on what may be a landmark study regarding hospice care. The study compared the quality of life and length of life for people who chose to use hospice and those who did not. The result was that people who used hospice lived longer and had better self-reported quality of life than those who did not use it.[5]

Hospice care during the last months of life is far less expensive than curative or the typical path of "doing everything" to stay alive. People qualify for hospice only after receiving a medical diagnosis of a terminal life span due to a specific disease, and a physician determines that the person is probably in the final six months of life. The person choosing hospice also agrees not to pursue further curative treatment, along with some other criteria. This is a decision made with health-care providers and the patient's closest loved ones, following good, objective advice, and is not solely a financial decision.

I bring up this topic because the surviving family members are affected in many ways (including finances), but so is society. And the social question is how dollars should best be used as people age. When in hospice, the elder receives treatment necessary for comfort and palliation of pain, in addition to social, spiritual, family, and other support. Many families report that, as difficult as death is to face, hospice provides support and help so that people can live with dignity, purpose, and compassion until they die. Hospice also offers continuing support to the bereaved person for a year after the loved one's death.

It is clear from research and practice that neither assertive curative treatment nor hospice services are intended to hasten death. The research results underscore the irony that aggressive curative treatment often brings more pain, inconvenience, and uncertainty than with hospice. It is unclear whether the assertive treatment causes people to have fewer days or if hospice causes them to live longer. In either case, the question is more one of what the elder's quality of life will be through the days that remain, and which is more desirable.

Small research studies in several retirement communities are suggesting that elders and their families more often choose hospice when they have a primary physician they know well, respect, and trust. This occurs when a trusted physician helps them objectively compare the facts of what their experience of assertive treatment is likely to be and what it realistically may achieve, compared with the experience of hospice and the managing of life and disease through an inevitable result. When elders can think through the various difficult scenarios with wise counselors, they can make informed choices. The experience in the retirement communities has been that increasing numbers of elders and their families are choosing the hospice option. This data requires more study but may provide a clue as to how to allocate funds regarding end-of-life care.

Application

"For the love of money is a root of all kinds of evil. Some people, eager for money, have wandered from the faith and pierced themselves with many griefs" (1 Tim. 6:10).

Few things can create disharmony in a family as money. Whether it is too little or a great amount is not relevant. How it is spent, who decides how the money is used, or who should or should not get it, and what they expect are all issues that must be addressed—all in consideration of the elder's needs. Families have split over money, and, in most cases, it is unnecessary. The person who made the money and controls it gets to make the decisions. The heirs should not consider it theirs until and if they receive any of it.

One of the best strategies for the use of money is to have a trusted, well-vetted financial advisor assisting the elder. If the person is a fiduciary and independent of the family, he or she is bound by law to take the elder's best interests in mind while being subject to the elder's wishes. A lawyer may also serve as the fiduciary and may be particularly helpful in the case of numerous family issues such as late-in-life second marriages, prenuptial arrangements, and other challenges.

Retirement communities come in a wide variety of sizes, types, and features. Each community has a different feel and way things occur. It is important to ensure that if one is chosen, it has the range of services to meet the desires of the elder today and the possible needs of the future. A good retirement community can increase the quality years of an older person. This can greatly benefit elders and their families.

Unscrupulous people are searching for older people they can steal from. Taking steps with an elder to help prevent a scam or theft can both reassure the elder and the family members. It is important that whoever is helping with the finances be completely transparent with the rest of the family to avoid issues of misbehavior.

Health-care costs at the end of life often are far more than people expect. What an heir might think is "his" may be needed for the health care of the elder. The assets should be used for the care of the elder.

When considering treatment later in life, it is good to understand how that will likely affect the elder's quality of life. While it is difficult to think of the last days of a beloved family member, be open and honest about talking with his or her health professional regarding the options. If it is appropriate, have the doctor introduce the concept of hospice to the elder and other family members. Choose a direction with care, filled with dialogue, thought, and prayer.

Takeaway Thoughts

How much money is enough? Money provides access to resources, but money itself does not add years or pleasure to life. It comes down to how the money should be used for the best outcome. The challenge is, who decides what the best outcome is: the elder, the family, or the government?

Many older people have a strong desire that they should pass money on to the next generation. Having that mindset is not wrong, but it can lead to difficulties and conflicts within the family. Setting money aside for grandchildren's education can be most helpful. But when elders give up things they want to do or have to be able to pass on money to the family, they need to weigh the value of what they give up against the impact of the gift. At times families can use funds irresponsibly, expecting the parent's estate to pull them out of debt. The elder needs good counsel to decide how and why funds should be given away in a manner that the funds do the most good.

The term *retirement community* does not mean a nursing home. Several types of care and services for older people and multiple price ranges are available. Research suggests that people who move into communities for older people often have more years of independence than those who stay in their homes. This may be due to access to meals, medication, exercise, and socialization.

Long-term care insurance can be a helpful tool to protect an elder's assets in that the insurance reduces the rate of spending on nursing homes or assisted living. In some states, however, if one has long-term care insurance and not many other assets convertible to cash, it could render an elder ineligible for certain types of assistance. It is important to have an insurance agent who knows and understands long-term care and the state's rules if there is any risk of the elder running low on cash.

Some people intend to divert an older person's assets into unhealthy or unsafe arrangements. Some want to take the elder's money while others are not aware of the risk of loss for an elder. Younger people have time to rebuild their assets if they run into financial difficulties; elders do not have the luxury of time to work for them. It is important to use insight and wisdom to avoid scams and outright theft of funds. Some unsavory characters see older people as a storehouse of money just for the taking.

End-of-life care can be prohibitively expensive. Since no one knows when death will come, a great proportion of dollars are spent in the last year of a person's life. However, when curative measures will no longer cure, hospice has a record of providing more and better-quality last days than if it is not used.

Questions for Consideration

1. How much money do you think is enough for an elder to maintain his or her lifestyle?
2. What should you do if an elder you know is scammed or runs out of money?
3. What is your experience with end-of-life choices for an elder?
4. How would you feel if an elder you love had tens of thousands of dollars at the end of her or his life? And gave those funds to you? And gave those funds to charity or another family member? Would you change your attitude and behavior toward her now?
5. What would your response be if an elder used all his funds for vacations and trips?
6. What would your response be if she used all her funds for health care?
7. What are your feelings about hospice, and do you think it extends life? Explain your answer.

7

Preserving the Elder's Legacy

Relationships

In a morning Bible study, a man requested prayer for his home. His mother-in-law had moved in with his family and was causing great disruption. The woman's behavior was putting a wedge between him and his wife and creating issues with the kids. The mother-in-law was demeaning to his wife and expecting the family to care for all of her needs while inserting herself into the middle of daily life. Additionally, she corrected his wife's folding of clothes and "proper" cooking techniques. The strain was so great that it was triggering health issues for him. He and his wife were bickering and fighting like they never had during their entire forty-two-year marriage. The issues continue even though they had had frank discussions with his mother-in-law.

They were dealing with several complex issues, including the mother-in-law's need for significance and value, and co-opting the family's structure and dynamic. The man quoted 1 Timothy 5:8: "Anyone who does not provide for their relatives and especially their household, has denied the faith and is worse than an unbeliever." His struggle was how to deal with the mother-in-law without becoming sinful or being "worse than an unbeliever." Yet they could not continue to bear the strain that could cause the marriage to fail.

Many believers struggle with this verse in 1 Timothy. How do we maintain a viable relationship with God while positively and gracefully enduring painful relational difficulties with family members in need? This is even more difficult when children are present. How do we walk faithfully, modeling godly behavior and love to our children, in this kind of challenge? Is it possible to thrive in them? Scriptures have much to say regarding perseverance, endurance, and living through hard things in life. A library of material about this and the general topic is available, so we will not dive deep into it. However, we will explore a deeper understanding of this passage, shedding light on each person's role.

Background

"Listen to your father, who gave you life, and do not despise your mother when she is old" (Prov. 23:22).

During the last days of his life and ministry, Paul wrote letters to Timothy to instruct, encourage, and remind his "son in the faith" how to lead and structure the churches he was pastoring. Early in 1 Timothy, Paul wrote of God's grace that he experienced and reminded Timothy to hold fast to the gospel as well as instructed him in faith and guidance of prophecy. After setting that foundation, he taught Timothy on orderly worship and structuring the church with solid, qualified, and prepared leadership through elders and deacons. He reminded Timothy that there will be false teaching that added human rules and laws that can never improve the gospel. He also spoke of communicating respectfully to both older and younger men and women. In the context of keeping the gospel unencumbered and central in relating to others, Paul gave his son in the faith instructions specific to the treatment of widows.

As chapter 2 describes, in Paul's time, people lived to an older age, as they do today, though fewer made it to that age. The harshness of life and the lack of modern medicine meant that more marriages ended in a spouse's death. In the culture of the time, men were to continue working to care for their families and themselves ("retirement" is a modern convention). Women often did not earn a wage, or if they did, it was so low as not to sustain them. Without substantive wages, how were the women to survive when their husbands died? At that time, the society was a paternal, mostly agrarian society in which an individual family's economy was based on what could be grown, made, or bartered. The familial responsibility fell to the male or the oldest son, based on both the law and the culture of the time. Widows who had no family to support them could end up in deep poverty.

In that context, Paul instructed the younger women to work, marry, and have children. It was not that Paul held women in poor esteem or subjugation to men. But in that culture, marriage and children were the main way women were protected. Without retirement plans, Social Security, and other means, raising children, particularly males, meant that a family member was responsible to care for the widow in her older age. In a real sense, children could provide a widow's security in retirement. While this context is foreign to the twenty-first-century mindset, it is important to remember that a person without a family and community role to fill was very much on their own in this agrarian culture.

In the first century, people who became believers in Jesus were, ironically, considered godless. To the Jews, the believers in Christ trusted in an anathema. To the gentiles, they forsook the panoply of gods generally accepted in society. To be a believer often resulted in being cut off from family and shunned by the communities in which they spent their lives. Because the society was patriarchal, younger women whose husbands died could more easily remarry than the older widows, who were beyond childbearing and were considered "too old" to raise a family.

Paul asserted that believing and faithful widows over sixty with no children or relatives to care for them were to be cared for by the church. If an older widow had children, Paul instructed that the adult children should care for them. Those adult children who did not care for their mothers were worse than an unbeliever. That passage is, of course, why many believers struggle with caring for elders who are making life hard, especially when they are living under the same roof.

BOB BENSON

Understanding the Language

The key to understanding 1 Timothy 5:8 is in the Greek word often translated as "care." In our culture and time, this word implies that we are to do all that is necessary for the elder to live well, often bringing them into our homes. To do otherwise is at some level uncaring; often interpreted as morally wrong and sinful. However, the original Greek word does not imply that we are required to bring a frail elder with multiple comorbidities into our homes. While the Greek word can be adequately translated as "care," it can also be translated as "making provision for," "providing forethought for," "to be concerned about," or "to take thought for." According to *Kittles Theological Dictionary of the New Testament*, the Greek word refers to making any kind of provision for and not just meeting a legal requirement as an heir would. Another translation of the word can be "give regard for," as in 2 Corinthians 8:21 and Romans 12:17. The *Septuagint* uses the same word in Proverbs 3:4: "Then you will win favor [good regard] and a good name in the sight of God and man."

What does it mean to make provision for or to have regard for an elder? It can mean bringing someone into your home. It can also mean building a mother-in-law home adjacent to your home or next door. Making provision for or regarding someone's interests is to make sure she has a roof over her head, she is safe, and her needs met. We must be thoughtful to interpret the Scriptures' translations as the words are used and contextually intended. An example of this is Paul's exhortation to Timothy to drink a little wine for his stomach. It is not clear, but Paul may have been referring to a detail specific to Timothy rather than giving us the go-ahead to drink a glass of wine whenever we have heartburn.

Understanding the nature of the word translated as "care," meaning to give regard for or be concerned about, is important in this context. This passage is not instructing us to move Maleficent the Mother-in-Law into our homes. It means we need to make sure that the elders we are responsible for have all they need for life and health. This can include their living in another town, where they are comfortable and safe, and ensuring that their needs are met. The

140

central theme is that they are cared about in such a way that the family plans for and makes meaningful provisions for the older woman. That provision can be in a believer's home, in the widow's longtime home with support, or in a care arrangement such as an apartment, assisted living, or even a nursing home if needed.

The language of 1 Timothy 5:8 means that arrangements for an elder should be made to benefit the widow. For example, a family can arrange for home care workers to look after an elder following surgery or to take care of other needs that arise. It also means that the elder can move into assisted living or a nursing home if necessary. The responsibility believers have toward their loved ones is to ensure that their situations are made with forethought and due regard for their best interest as a valued member of the family. The greater message through Scripture is to consider other people's needs before your own. Do what you can to help.

It is common for a family to feel guilty about placing a loved one in any kind of care setting, or they experience guilt for feeling "put out" when they bring an elderly loved one into their homes. Somehow, we can feel that we have let them down or given up on them and that we should not feel that way. In God's merciful nature, he does not judge us for not having the resources to care for a loved one. Instead, we are to take thought, plan, and do what we can for the elderly loved one. The guilt families feel comes from expectations we have of ourselves or that the elder may place on us.

One definition of being overwhelmed is when our resources and abilities are insufficient to handle whatever circumstances we face. We can feel overwhelmed when caring for an older person, particularly when our emotional, physical, financial, and time resources run thin. Responsible provision for the elder is through using the means we have with integrity to our best ability. Taking that responsibility to heart implies that we will seek appropriate help in caring for an older family member. This approach is healthy.

Feeling guilty for the inability to give physical, emotional, or financial aid is not a helpful or healthy way to cope. Ask for help in dealing with the guilt, or look for a support group to assist. It can greatly improve the relationship with the elder and the advocate's other relationships. First Timothy 5:8 is not written to induce guilt; rather, it clarifies for whom we are to take particular concern: the widow, in this case. Elsewhere it is the widow and the orphan (James 1:27) and the poor (Proverbs 31:9, Luke 14:14).

Some elders will play the guilt card. Realize, though, that providing hands-on, emotional, or cognitive care for another person twenty-four hours a day seven days a week is hard, exhausting work, particularly when family support is limited or when the caregiver is also elderly. Getting help can be a good thing for sustaining the caregiver's and care receiver's emotional states and health. Each year nursing homes have "double admissions" when an unpaid caregiver, often a spouse, is worn down and falls or has medical needs of her own. Both caregiver and care receiver are admitted for care and support at the same time. It is better if the caregiver can provide support for an elder without having to do all the work herself. This puts the caregiver in a better position to ensure proper regard for and protection of the elder while keeping her own health intact.

Often an older caregiver feels it is her or his duty from the marriage vows to continue caring for the spouse at home. Sometimes spouses (especially men) convince their mates that they must care for them at home until "death does them part." Again, while it is thought to be a loving and committed thing to do, make sure the physical and emotional cost to the caregiver does not erode the relationship or make the caring one directional. The one who receives care may not be taking the caregiver's interest as more important than his own and may reflect fear, selfishness, or pride. Absolutely nothing is wrong with providing hands-on care to a spouse as he needs it. The issue to watch for is if the caregiving extends for such a time that it draws down the physical and emotional resources of the caregiver, erodes the relationship, or both. Getting help is vital to sustaining the relationship, whether it comes through a family member, friend, home care worker, adult day center, or full-time placement in an alternative setting. Do not forget that the spouse or close family member can provide the love, support, and legacy as no outside person can. Others can provide hands-on care, but they can never replace that individual and personal connection to loved ones. It is important to retain that key relationship.

Abuse and Neglect

Much has been said about the abuse and neglect of elders. The Scriptures speak clearly against such practices. It needs to be said, though, that unintentional (or intentional) abuse or neglect can occur when a caregiver is overtired and does not have the stamina for long-term care without support. Weariness and frustration can increase to the point where unintended harm can occur. People need to be particularly wary when the elder needing care has significant cognitive decline. Repeated questions or comments all day long or the risk of wandering out of the home and getting lost causes immense stress for the caregiver. At times people with cognitive issues can become combative due to frustration, lack of understanding and being understood, or other reasons, and the caregiver might be harmed as well. Safety and protection for all people in the household are paramount. Resources and support groups are available to assist and educate caregivers and are highly recommended. Groups dedicated to Alzheimer's disease, Parkinson's, and many other syndromes and conditions are available. Usually, a primary care physician or a social worker can help a caregiver and their family find a group that can provide support, education, and resources.

Abuse can be physical, emotional, or verbal. Anything that is threatening the health and well-being of a frail elder should be considered abuse and needs to be reported.

Neglect is the withholding of necessary care or services that could also threaten the health and well-being of an elder. If abuse or neglect is suspected, contact the local law enforcement or adult protective services. If unsure how to proceed, contact the patient's primary care provider or social worker.

Relational Foundations

The fifth commandment is listed twice in the Old Testament: "Honor thy father and your mother, as the Lord your God has commanded you, so that you may live long and that it may go well with you in the land the Lord your God is giving you" (Deut. 5:16); and "Honor your father and your mother, so that you may live long in the land the Lord your God is giving you" (Exod. 20:12).

God wrote the Ten Commandments on slabs of stone (twice), which Moses subsequently carried down the mountain to the people of Israel. These commands were part of the foundation for what was later to come: the law. As Christians, we are free from the Levitical law, but it can be argued that we are compelled even more to love God and our neighbors as ourselves—and doing so perfectly would complete the requirements of the law. But to do so, we would have to be God. Of course, we all fail to love God with all our hearts, souls, minds, and strength, and we fall far short of loving our neighbors as ourselves. We need Jesus to complete or fulfill the law's requirements for us. So then, relative to the fifth commandment, does it apply to us in our consideration of aging? If so, how?

In Sunday school, most kids had to memorize the Ten Commandments, and then in vacation Bible school we went over them again (with crafts!), and finally in confirmation (Lutheran catechism), we had to memorize them yet again along with Luther's understanding: "What does this mean?" There must be a reason for children to learn and study the commandments multiple times. They do, or at least did, inform our Judeo-Christian moral basis. As for the fifth commandment, if we did not obey our parents, were we destined to a short life ending in a fiery death while working on our driver's permits?

The moral teaching of the Ten Commandments is important as a basis for our culture and society. It is instructive for children to learn and, as is the case for any Scripture, for anyone to meditate upon. But the fifth commandment can pose problems with its understanding and application. When I was a youngster attending Sunday school, one of the more worldly students asked the teacher,

"What happens to the promise of a long life if your parents tell you to break one of the other commandments and you don't do it?" After fumbling a bit, she said that the pastor would be discussing that in detail during confirmation classes…when we were older. She then said that in general, if our parents told us to break one of the commandments, we did not have to honor that request.

Does the ancient fifth commandment hold any promise for us today, particularly as we age? Note that the "you" in the fifth commandment is a plural "you," meaning all of you together as a nation or society. This is an important distinction because if society as a whole respects parental authority (even the "bad" parents) as well as people in other types of authority, the society can address adult concerns and right its wrongs. Yes, this is an aspirational statement, but that does not invalidate the premise. It is a commandment to which we can aspire but cannot perfectly reach.

Growing up in a small town in Minnesota, I lived for a time on the wrong side of the railroad tracks. My brother and I were reasonably responsive to our parents' dictates. When my older brother and I were new to town, just entering seventh and eighth grade, we each experienced "bad" through no fault of our own. Living on the "North Side" meant that for the first time we had to ride the bus to school. Two guys, the local bullies shared our bus stop. They started sitting in the bus seat behind my brother and me every day to and from school. They would do everything junior high tormentors did: slap us, make us drop books, berate us, call us names, light my brother's hair on fire, stick gum in our hair…You get the picture. We tried to sit in front of a group of girls every chance we got.

One afternoon, the bullies got behind us and were especially threatening. They began bragging to the others on the bus about how they were going to beat us up. As we stood to get off the bus, the bigger of the two hit my brother in the ear, which began to swell at once, and bent his glasses. All of the kids unloaded from the bus at our stop to see the fight, which was sure to be brutal. Somehow, my brother and I walked through the crowd and went home to the hoots and howls of our cowardice from the riled group. We thought we were going to be chased down and decimated, but the bullies stayed in their little knot of kids and then went home. They did not bother us much after that except when one of them sucker-punched me before school. I could not breathe and thought I would asphyxiate, but that was the last of the bullying. Fast-forward about twenty years. I was back in that little town. I ran into an old friend and asked what happened to the bully who sucker-punched me. My friend said that he had died in prison.

The problem with the bullies was not the disaffection for my brother and me. We survived and can tell the story. The relevance of the story is that I know now that neither of the two tough guys respected their teachers, parents, other people, or peers. The issues created by and through their disrespect for others resulted in a short-ened life for at least one, if not both. No doubt there were surely other issues at play in their lives, but the example is real. The conse-quence for that young man was a shortened life. It does not always happen that way—Psalms are full of wicked people who live long and prosper while righteous people are poor and die early. As a society, though, the ideal of respecting authority is foundational to helping improve the culture and general life experience.

The fifth commandment is certainly about respecting parents, and in the broader sense, it is about respecting authority—even human authority. Think about how the Israelites identified them-selves as the children of Israel. They called Abraham, Isaac, and Jacob their fathers just as we call God our Father. Lack of respect for the fathers in that environment meant disrespect of their culture, peo-ple, God, and the law—everything that defined them. The fifth commandment then and now relates to the core of who we are as believers.

However, what if the authorities over us do not abide by our same principles? Does the fifth commandment still apply? Scriptures cite some notable pre-law examples demonstrating respect: after Abram rescued Lot, his family, and his possessions from capture, he gave ten percent of his plunder to Melchizedek, the Priest King of Salem (Gen. 14:17–24). Jacob worked for twenty years for Laban, treating Laban's goods as more important than his, though he did not trust Laban (Gen. 29:14–30, 31:38–42). Post-law examples include Daniel working in high positions for three nations' kings, none of whom respected or followed Jewish law. Samuel obeyed Eli, whose sons had no regard for the Lord (1 Sam. 2:12, 26). After Saul attempted to kill David more than once, David spared Saul's life (1 Sam. 26:7–25). Additional Old Testament examples demonstrate the prophets and others who respected authorities God had placed over them, though they often spoke God's harsh but true words to teach the authorities to turn back to God.

The New Testament provides examples of submitting to unbelieving authorities. Think about how Paul appealed to Caesar (who considered himself a deity). How it was prophesied that Peter would one day be shackled and led away to his death. The ultimate example is Jesus, who went before the authorities as a lamb to the slaughter. When Jesus was being betrayed, he knew what was happening and did not strike out or try to talk his way out of his coming punishment (John 18:4–9). (Though he demonstrated his authority when the arresting group drew away from him and fell to the ground when he said, "I am he" [John 18:5].) Even in the trial before the Sanhedrin, Jesus spoke respectfully (Matt. 26:62–66, John 18:19–24).

There is more to consider, though. A subtle reality is tucked within the fifth commandment: "that it may go well with you." This is not a patent guarantee that a long, happy life will happen for those who obey their parents. The Ten Commandments were given to a nation, not just individuals. In that sense, the promise applies to a cohort or nation of people. As an individual experience, some people who obeyed their parents died early. Conversely, some who greatly disobeyed their parents lived long, rich lives. The subtlety's relevance is that children simultaneously age at the same rate as their parents. In that process, we all transition both into our personalities and roles relative to one another.

Sometimes an adult caregiver will remark that she has become the parent and the parent has become the child, such as being unable to make decisions. This ever-transitioning relationship as we age is key to the "may go well with you" phrase of the fifth commandment. One truth in life is that we bring our relationships with our parents, grandparents, and siblings into our adult lives. Learning how to respect, honor, healthily conflict and love our family helps create good relationships. Healthy relationships guide children and parents through a successful aging experience. This is what "it may go well with you" looks like.

Children bring their historic relationships with their parents and siblings into a simultaneous aging process and experience. How mature the individuals are is just one factor. The relationships are usually exacerbated by the years of previous experience together. If a family's children and parents have a warm, supportive relationship through adulthood, when a crisis occurs, that behavior tends to continue. However, if the relationship has been tumultuous, the same crises that will bring some families closer together can decimate another family's tenuous relationships.

The status of the sibling relationship can often be seen when decisions must be made for the parents' care when crises occur. Typically, gender and birth order return—the historic relationships and roles of the children come into play. In the US, it is common to see the oldest female child stepping into the responsibility of caring for the parents. If the parents had no female children, often the spouse of the eldest son ends up carrying the load. As in any generality, there are exceptions to this observation, but it is a frequent order of relationship even when the parent and the eldest female do not get along.

Ironically, the training and profession of each child may not be relevant, depending on how well the siblings work together for common good. My eldest sister became the caregiver and coordinator of our parents' care. She handled the role beautifully with the support of her younger sister, a physician, and our youngest brother, who had been serving in aging services for years. My older brother has the least training and exposure in health care, but he had insights and asked valuable questions that were most helpful. It was clear to me where I fit in the decision-making process and how I could help. We knew our positions in the family order and used those traditional places to the advantage of our parents. I am proud of how my sisters and brothers worked through the difficulties of health issues and the frailty of our parents.

A common source of conflict occurs between the siblings who are with the elder frequently and those who are not as involved. This is especially the case when one or more of the siblings live hours away. Often, less-involved or distant children see the aging parent and family challenges differently than the ones who are there frequently. It is not necessarily a lack of concern or love; rather, it is more likely that the distant sibling's face-to-face experience with the parent is not the same. When we speak on the phone or a video message, we often portray our best selves, or at least only a part of ourselves. The disadvantage of telecommunications is that we cannot observe the daily behavior of the person on the other end of the line. Mom may be dressed and have her hair combed but not have adequate food in the refrigerator; she may be cutting medications in half to save cost or be unsteady in how she walks—a fall waiting to happen.

Being with a parent allows the nearby child to note how life is for the elder and may call out a concern. The distant sibling cannot see the problems and may diminish the level of the issue's relevance. The closer sibling may start emphasizing the risks more energetically. The distant sibling then attempts to connect more with the parent yet remains unable to see the issue. A circular dance ensues, the one sibling escalating an alarm and the other diminishing its presence... until a crisis occurs with the parent. Then both siblings respond with guilt and anger (for different reasons) toward each other. This conflict between the responsiveness of the siblings compounds the parent's crisis. Just when the siblings need to pull together, their relationship, cracked from prior years of differences, can fracture. The answer is to work hard at the communication between the siblings and encourage the distant one to spend significant time with the parent at risk, if possible.

"That it may go well with you" is found in how respect is displayed among the family members. It is important that things go well during crises. Working together as a family team greatly increases the chances for good outcomes for the one needing care. It also opens the possibility for the siblings to redirect their relationships. Parents are not oblivious to fractured relationships in the family and between the children. When the parent is in a crisis and the tension between siblings increases, it causes added stress for the parent, who needs support.

It can be tempting for adult children to treat parents as children, particularly if cognitive decline occurs. Significantly, our parents do not become children, though they may have childlike behavior or be unable to grasp the realities of their situation. They are adults needing help, a vastly different proposition from caring for children. Even in severe cognitive loss, older people, who may not recognize their children or spouses, still respond to kindness. If there is minimal cognitive loss, we may not agree with our older loved ones' decisions or life choices, but they usually recognize when people are being calm and caring with them. The aging are adults, and they tend to do better when they have real choices, even if those choices must be simplified and they do not like the nature of the options. Many older people have all of their faculties and still make decisions the family may not agree with. So long as they understand the consequences of their decisions, they are the decision makers.

In some cases, there may be opportunities to deepen and strengthen the relationship with an aging parent. While we reside in the same bodies we have had since birth, who we are sixty, seventy, or eighty years are not exactly who we were in our twenties and thirties. Time and experience ameliorate who we become. With years and different perspectives honed through experience, the chance to reestablish or deepen familial relationships may open. Approaching relationships with the knowledge that perspectives and realities are different today than decades earlier may give opportunities to see parents in a new light. There is a risk of trying to put a relationship to rest after years of difficulty. However, in and after a crisis, relationships and needs can change and could create an opportunity for meaningful dialogue.

Since we bring our existing family relationships into our aging parents' issues, how can we navigate decisions if there are years of differences and acrimony with the parents or siblings? Consider trying to call a truce. What that means is to acknowledge that each person's hurt feelings, questioned motives, actions, and interpretations exist and that the past can make a current situation harder to work through. At times, asking for a truce on those emotions and memories may work. I do not mean to deny them but, rather, to recognize them and ask all to set them aside for an important time. The adult focus should be on the elder in crisis, and all voices are needed to participate meaningfully for the best interests of the person in crisis. Not attempting to give and hear everyone's opinions can lead to conflict during and after the crisis. Ensure that each voice is acknowledged, though not every opinion needs to be followed. This is not an easy time for anyone, regardless of the relational status between all people involved, but an elder at risk needs singular focus and common support. The ideal is if everyone can discuss and agree to whatever plan is necessary for the at-risk elder's safety and care. If all cannot agree on a solution, turn to an independent person for counsel or advice. This could be a physician, social worker, pastor, or other respected individuals.

Finally, on the fifth commandment, if possible, invite all those influencing the decisions into the dialogue. It may be a difficult experience, but in the long run, it is often the best. This is for two main reasons. First, getting everyone involved to understand the facts of the issue/crisis is necessary to come to any agreement regarding care and services needed. Second, some family members possess knowledge, resources, and understanding that might shed surprising light on the situation. Other voices might even propose a creative solution to a difficult situation. Always remember that, as much as possible, the adult receiving care also needs a voice in this process. Research is clear that an elder who decides or at least participates in a difficult decision has a much greater likelihood of doing better with that decision. Ultimately, that approach respects all participants, laying a foundation for improving relationships through the family. Then that goal of communication and dialogue can help make things "go well with you."

Relational Expectations

There once was a young fellow starting his career working for a national company serving almost all fifty states. The head of Human

Resources asked him where he thought his first placement as a man-
ager would be. After thinking a moment, the young man replied,
"Pump Handle, North Dakota." (A town that does not exist.)
Surprised, the older man asked him why he expected an assignment
there. "Because if you send me there, it's what I expect, and if you
don't, I will be grateful."

Much of our lives are driven by expectations and our perspectives of those expectations. Many people in their nineties say that
they never expected to live that long. People in their teens never really
expect to get old. The reality is that aging impacts our expectations
and perspectives while coloring our future experiences.

As each of us ages, our relationships age with us. Our future
changes by how we nurture those relationships. We may see the effect
of relational developments as we age. What we may not see are the
expectations we carry about those relationships. Comments like, "I
always thought she would be with us" or "He died too young" are
common at funerals and gatherings. When a sudden death ends a
relationship, we often express shock and briefly recognize life's brev-
ity. The writer of Ecclesiastes encourages us to number our days and
recognize that the silver cord of our lives has a specific length (Eccles.
12:6–7). Psalms and Proverbs also teach us to number our days. The
truth is, the longer we live, the more people we will know who pass
out of our lives. An older woman once said, "Why is it that I live,
and all my friends and family have died?" One person described getting older as being at a train station with all his friends and family.
Everyone else gets on board the trains that come and go. You notice
it at first and wave them off until suddenly, you stand alone, waiting
for your train.

For many, the loss of old friends and family is not only the
death of a relationship but also the loss of either a shared history
experienced together or living a history yet hoped for. Each of us
is aware of special times with a friend that will pass from shared to
solitary if that friend dies. It is important to remember that isolated
memories come alive when the events are shared with others. That
may be one reason why it is important to ask about and listen to the
stories elders share. Often their tales carry implicit wisdom, but the

telling is also the elder reexperiencing something that may live solely in his or her mind.

How does this knowledge help us to set expectations regarding aging? People feel regarded when others listen to their stories and even more if something is learned in the sharing. We should expect and ask elders to regale us with their histories. If they seem to repeat a certain story (or trauma) often, they may have been more emotionally impacted by the event and are still working with the story's wonder or struggle. To hear different stories, ask questions that will make them think of and relate other events in their lives. These questions both affirm the elder and help us learn.

Beyond the private histories, what do our expectations lead us to in working with elders? People assume a great many things about elders that are not necessarily true, such as believing that older people are physically or emotionally weak, they cannot understand technology, they are not mentally aware, etc. Other expectations we have of older people may cause serious issues. We might think they cannot understand a course of treatment, what is going on, or that their response to a given situation is out of proportion.

Promises made in the past regarding the elder create difficulties in the present. Time and again, children promise their parents never to place Mom or Dad in a nursing home. The issue comes about when the care needs of the elder overwhelm the child's or children's ability to provide the necessary care. This causes issues within the family: increasing guilt and opposing viewpoints about what to do. When an elder has a significant, sudden health event requiring quick life-changing decisions, the earlier promises, which were made in the absence of context, become barriers to considering options and opportunities for care. Parental or spousal expectations like this can drive wedges between family members, sometimes affecting the rest of their relationships.

A similar expectation occurs when a person promises themselves that they will never place their parent somewhere for twenty-four-hour care. Some realities make this an unrealistic expectation. These promises, though made with good intent, may not be consistent with a future crisis. This is like having a child who decides and expects not to ever have a cavity. The child does not control all the variables and sets himself up for disappointment if he or she ends up with a cavity. Promises do not control future variables in an elder's life. Promises today cannot accurately reflect care options not yet developed today but will be available when a specific need arises. If there is a promise to be made, make the one that says, "We will make certain to watch for your best interests always."

Parents' money and estates can create expectations, pressure, and discord in decisions for spending their money. Many elders promise themselves and their families to leave money in their estates. In those cases, it becomes much harder for elders to use their money for fun, care, or needed services. If we look at our parents' money through selfishness or greed, we may create deep and lasting rifts in our families and with our parents. Expecting our parents' wealth to solve our personal financial difficulties when they die may be like relying on the wind. The last year of life can have huge medical and other expenses. If a nursing home or at-home care is required for any significant time, the drain on the estate will be large. An elder does not have to share the contents of their wills before they die, and they can change them at any time. The point is that we cannot expect our parents' estates to give us a boost in our financial situations. There might not be any money left, and if there is, expectations can cause all sorts of legal and financial issues for the family. It is best to encourage elders to use the funds as they see fit, and if there is an estate, great, but it is to be an appreciated gift in any amount or thought. Wisdom of the Scripture addresses this:

- The righteousness of the upright delivers them, but the unfaithful are trapped by evil desires. (Prov. 11:6)
- Whoever seeks good finds favor, but evil comes to the one who searches for it. Those who trust in riches will fall, but the righteous will thrive like a green leaf. (Prov. 11:27–28)
- Better is a little with righteousness than much gain with injustice. (Prov. 16:8)

- Do not wear yourself out to get rich; do not trust your own cleverness. Cast but a glance at riches, and they are gone, for they will surely sprout wings and fly off to the sky like an eagle. (Prov. 23:4–5)
- An inheritance gained too soon will not be blessed in the end. (Prov. 20:21)

All concerned should set aside expectations of the future and place the future in God's hands. Acknowledge the selfishness we all have, look to the best interest of the elders in our lives, and help others to do so as well. The money our parents earned is theirs to do with as they wish. Serve the parents with love for their best interests. No money can equal serving others with integrity.

Application

This chapter focused on how aging people can create unique challenges and problems in the family. We explored what the Scriptures teach on caring for family members in our homes and how can they inform discussions in difficult family dynamics with both believers and unbelievers. The intent was not to answer the specific issues in detail but to provide a scriptural framework from which elder care can be viewed as it relates to the family.

The Scriptures call us to care for family members by making provision for them as they need. This is not a requirement to move them into our homes; rather, we are to ensure they have proper care and protection.

One important key in helping older people is to listen and understand their perspectives and do all we can to protect the relationship. That is because no friend or acquaintance can replace family relationships. That means enlisting the support of other caregivers and health professionals to assist as needed. It could even mean being the "bad guy" while making the best decisions.

The fifth commandment tells us to honor our parents. It does not require anyone to like each other, but the Scriptures do say to consider others' needs as more important than our own. When helping an older family member, this is helpful guidance. It is especially helpful when members of the family dispute what is best for the elder. Maintaining focus on what is best for the elder first may help avoid some issues.

When an elder has a crisis and needs family support, the nature of the family dynamic joins into that crisis. For example, it is common for the family birth order to have a role as does any simmering or outright unresolved conflicts between the siblings or the aging person. It is ideal if the family discusses what to do before any crisis occurs, but that is not always possible. Declaring a truce to focus on the issue at hand may help. It is necessary to keep the person in crisis in the center of focus, not the other interpersonal issues. Work hard for the benefit of the one needing help with as much openness and transparency as possible.

In a difficult family crisis, consider how the situation may help build bridges between people in conflict. By working together, opportunities may open for a new level of listening and dialogue. While there is no guarantee, one person once said, "Let's not allow a crisis go to waste."

Takeaway Thoughts

God created families for many reasons. One is that he designed families as an instant community for every person. The passage in 1 Timothy 5 provides a glimpse of how families were designed to work. We do have a responsibility toward one another, particularly if no one else is there to provide care. It does not mean that outside resources cannot be used if needed.

The fifth commandment offers further guidance on how families are designed to work. However, the context is critical in understanding the command. The commandment is given to the plural "you" and applied to Israel as a nation. Children need to learn obedience to parents and transmute that understanding to adults who need to respect authority, as the Scriptures declare. It does not mean that if William disobeys his mom, he will die early. But if an entire nation of Williams does not respect authority, anarchy is waiting at that country's door. We are responsible to apply the commandment individually so that a nation of Williams does not occur. Note that the commandment does not end when the child becomes an adult. Nor does it require blind obedience to the parent. Respectfully considering the other person's best interest generally applies whether agreeing with them or not.

Abuse and neglect do happen in families. Physical, verbal, emotional, and neglect abuse of elders is often hidden in the family context and comes to light in a crisis. Theft of an elder's assets is a form of abuse and is often seen by children collecting parents' retirement payments or "borrowing" money and never intending to pay it back.

We told our children that they must work and play together so they would always have playmates. We also said that family is for life, and the members can be lifelong support and encouragement for one another. They can also be gut-wrenching rivals for life. When an elder needs help or is in a crisis, the entire family offers their opinions on the solution. Even when siblings or others in the family conflict, navigating those waters early can save a great deal of hardship and conflict.

Sibling relationships affect the care and treatment of the elder family members. A parent's crisis is one time when factions need to set aside their disputes for the good of the family. An outside person may be able to help so long as they are viewed as independent of all parties.

Questions for Consideration

1. What is your perspective of 1 Timothy 5:8? Has the author's explanation of the verse caused a change in how you think of your responsibility toward others?
2. The fifth commandment is the first commandment with a promise. Is it difficult for you to honor your parents or one of your parents? Why? What can you do about that?
3. Does the deeper level of "that it may go well with you" make sense, and is it real?

4. Family relationships are often hard, carrying years of burdens and differences. Can you see how you might call a truce to those issues to focus on a parent at risk?
5. Is it honestly possible to use a crisis with a family member as an opportunity to restore relationships?
6. How might respect and engaging the sibling's input on decisions regarding a parent's care help to diminish conflict over a parent's estate?

8

Putting It Together

Boiling It Down

In this chapter, we will summarize the discussion of relevant portions of Scripture, how we might consider the wisdom of God's design of aging, and how we might look forward to and enjoy aging as the gift he bestows.

This book explored six general aspects of aging. The first two chapters discussed the Bible's distinct perspective of aging. We were designed by God to age. And in that design, the aged were to be respected. For example, the young were instructed to stand up in the presence of an older person. Our cultural perspectives of life expectancy and aging do not see aging in the same light as the Scripture portrays. Today, the term *senator* may no longer connote respect, but the Bible writers used respectful words to describe or address elders, the downcast, and the poor. Ours is a culture marginalizing, or treating as invisible, those who are not youthful or strong.

The American social structure did not put the aged, infirm, and poor as a social priority until President Lyndon Johnson's Great Society in the mid-1960s, nearly 180 years after the Philadelphia Constitutional Congress formally adopted the Constitution. Those social programs included Civil Rights, Medicare, and Medicaid. Before then there was not a codified system protecting our country's most vulnerable. Contrast the 180-year absence of US protections with the designs God's law implemented to benefit the aging. Beginning with the Ten Commandments given to Moses at Mt. Sinai, God established social structures demonstrating his compassion, mercy, and provision for the aged, infirm, and poor. God's grace and mercy are evident in how he perceived, protected, and provided for the aged from day one.

The law encouraged family strength and purposeful roles for all members of the family and provided respect for the elders in decision-making and community activity. The legal structures God set up uniquely included implicit means for those who had lost their land and were in poverty to regain the land after a time. The series of Jewish festivals and celebrations set at regular intervals were to ensure the return of land, fair trade, and reasonable rates of interest. All these things were to help ensure prosperity and provide social safety nets assisting all, especially the aged, infirm, and poor.

The third chapter considered how God provides special gifts we might apprehend as we age. In our culture, we do not look at the aging process as a time of special gifting and growth. Instead, the aged often feel overlooked or even invisible. This chapter considered several gifts that come through aging and how they might affect elders and those around them.

Some of the gifts are obvious, such as gaining experience over the years and the possibility of becoming wise. Other gifts, such as courage, frankness, and humility, as well as not feeling our age or how our emotions may grow or change by our experiencing years, may be less familiar to the reader. Recognizing and leveraging the gifts is an important tool in understanding and relating to elders while helping them to succeed in their purpose of loving God and enjoying him forever. In the mellowing of years, we often become more resolute with what is important and less so regarding secondary matters. As the Teacher and the psalms encourage us, we would do well to consider our own aging and how we might help others through our years.

Chapter 4 names a key element in serving elders well: becoming their advocate. Life transitions of any type go better when another person advocates your best interests along with you. The Scriptures are replete with examples of advocating for others and point to the work of Jesus and his advocacy for us. A common theme in advocacy though is it has an emotional cost and sometimes financial and physical cost too. Advocates benefit both the elders and themselves by seeking to understand the perspective of aging people and then work to support them. Several examples were supplied to illustrate how family members advocated for the elders in their lives.

The difficult issue of when the elder refuses care or does not allow the family to have information or voice can be breached through good advocacy in time. Yes, frustrating and maddening, but maintaining the role of an advocate through an elder's refusals can either show the advocate why the refusal is happening or make him or her a trusted helper when an incident or issue occurs. An advocate is a support, not the boss.

When does an advocate take charge of a situation? The general answer is it is best when the senior comes to his own decision. However, in the case where the life or safety of the elder or others is endangered, stepping in is warranted. There are consequences for when an advocate steps in and makes decisions for another person. They can include working through the elder's anger up to and including the breaking of the relationship. Loss of the advocate role does not have to be permanent, but even with love and good conflict resolution skills, the relationship may not be quite the same again.

Technology can aid both the elder and the advocate. New technologies supporting the independence of elders are becoming more common. With the arrival of the "internet of things," new ideas and helps are often coming on the market. The way to think about technology is that it is simply a tool. When an elder has an issue or behavior that is concerning, the advocate can go to the internet and search for solutions to that challenge. For example, if an elder has trouble sleeping and gets up at night, installing motion sensor night-lights that illuminate a path to the bathroom or other rooms is helpful. They typically use little energy and create enough light to see a path but not blind or startle the person with a bright light. Other devices can track a vehicle to ensure that the older parent is going where he or she ought to and is not in trouble. Technology stores and security plans often have inobtrusive devices and systems that can meet a particular need to assure advocates that their loved ones are protected and well. Naturally, these devices are purchased with the elders' knowledge and placed in ways to ensure their dignity. Advocates can use them as tools to help elders meet their goal of remaining independent and safe.

Chapter 5 showed that as we age, we are in constant transition in ourselves and in relation to others. We touched on the challenge of comorbidities—the simultaneous multiple syndromes and chronic ailments experienced by the aging—and how the treatment of one issue can exacerbate a separate issue. It is often the physical needs of aging that older people and their families must respond to and struggle with. The cognitive and emotional needs are significant, though less recognized or understood by families.

The challenges listed are not intended to be all-inclusive or to provide medical or legal advice; rather, they focus on topics not frequently regarded from a biblical point of view, though other literature or guides are available that might help.

Identifying what the aging are experiencing in their homes is critical to providing meaningful support and care. Many elderly people have significant limitations in their ability to perform basic tasks around the home. There are workarounds that, with the right advice and tools, can greatly improve the daily experiences of people who find some tasks difficult. Figuring out what older people need to live well takes a certain amount of attention to their environments, health, and what they are "giving up" because they cannot do them anymore. Casting a blind eye to these cues can mean an elder's increasing and faster decline. Likewise, it is possible to help too much, which results in gradually escalating their dependency and loss of function. Professionals can assist the aging in maximizing life quality, but the first line of defense is an attentive, informed, and honest appraisal of how well an elder is doing.

The remaining chapters addressed some of the financial, relational, mental, spiritual, and emotional aspects of aging.

Chapter 6 noted that many experts expound on what to do with money, often implying that the of measure life may be the size of a portfolio or bank account. This chapter reviewed aspects of aging with a perspective on money. We discussed the purpose and focus of an elder's funds. Money creates resources and options for the elder's care. The more resources we can apply to a situation, the more options appear. The internet is replete with advice on "how much money a retiree needs." In the years nearing retirement age, it is common for the aging to question and worry if they have enough funds to live well into their older years.

Jesus warns us about greed and told a parable about a rich fool who has much and builds barns to store more, yet his life is required of him that night (Luke 12:13–21). Jesus's analysis is "This is how it will be with whoever stores up things for themselves but is not rich toward God" (v. 21). Jesus made it clear that life is not made of how much we have. Unfortunately, money is an area where selfishness and greed can become all too apparent. Rather than focusing on what a person can gain from a parent's estate, the Scriptures encourage us to concentrate on treasures in heaven; this is key in how we handle our relationships.

Regarding finances and the use of money in aging, Scripture guides us from several different moral and ethical angles. Consider how God's law set up social structures and the value of relationships between him as well as the aging, infirm, and poor. From the very beginning of how we can live in reverence to God, we are instructed on the value of life over all else. In the Sermon on the Mount, Jesus speaks of ensuring we have treasures in heaven. That does not mean we should not plan to care for our future needs and those of our families. First Timothy 5 tells us to take thought for widows (including the ones left in our homes when their husbands die).

It is good to plan and think ahead and prepare, but what money we or our relatives have is not to be our source of hope. God, Jesus, is our salvation and hope. We do what we can to live wisely while trusting God for all of it. Tomorrow is not guaranteed to any of us; therefore, we should prepare for both our spouses and our many years and health-care needs in aging, knowing that we may not be granted many days. After all, what benefit is there in gaining the whole world yet losing the soul?

Consider taking the perspective that since the money elders have is theirs, help them to use it for their benefit and as they choose. It is a gift from the Lord to enjoy and can be used to bless the elders and the Lord. Help the older person avoid scammers and the multiple cons that target the elderly. Take care with elders' funds for their benefit.

Taking a thoughtful view of our relatives' estates is wise. While we may expect to inherit a share in our parents' wealth at their passing, we are not absolved of preparing for our own aging, and not only financially but also physically and spiritually. And do not forget that even though money could be coming your way in an estate, you cannot know how much you will receive until after all of the legal proceedings are complete, debts paid (often significant amounts for end-of-life health care), other beneficiaries, taxes, etc. Economies have highs and lows; what can seem to be plenty for the barns may suddenly disappear. Do not consider the estate to be the hope for your future. Instead, live within your means, and if an estate comes your way, use the estate to build relationships within the family and others in ways that honor God. Use the money to best serve the Lord. If it is needed to pay down your debts, use it as a help and blessing. Then work to stay out of debt so you can be a greater benefit to others.

Chapter 7 focused on how aging family members can create unique challenges and problems in the home of family members. Paul's letter to Timothy speaks directly to how widows should be treated. Looking deeply into 1 Timothy 5:8, we read that Paul advises us to take thought of and consider the needs of our elders. We are to make provisions for them, but that does not mean they are required to move into an adult child's home. Making provisions means ensuring that elders have the care and services they need to be safe, healthy, and free to make decisions.

Caregivers for older people are often spouses. Twenty-four-hour provision of care to a frail person is exhausting and can lead to ill health for the caregiver. It is not wrong to use outside help or one of the various forms of institutional care to serve an elder's needs. Using institutional help can, however, be a source of conflict and guilt for family members. Rather than perceiving this kind of help as "giving up," it is better to reframe the decision as ensuring that the frail person receives professional help so the family can focus on the emotional and spiritual support only the family can provide.

It is my hope that this chapter illustrates some challenges families face and reflects biblical truths, supplying new perspectives. Families may be able to heal some of the nagging relational issues they have because of the difficulties they encounter together. Crisis brings families together, giving new opportunities to set aside former patterns of behavior and to adopt Christ's humility, grace, and patience in the midst. This is not to imply that taking the attitude of Christ either diminishes the difficulty or solves it; rather, it is a way for those taking this path to behave with integrity and care. Healing has and can come through difficulties if families work through them together. As someone once said, "It would be a shame to waste a good crisis."

The Scriptures teach about caring for family members, and they inform discussions families can have about the elder's needed care and decisions that go along with it. The perspectives of Scripture can help with difficult family dynamics that include both believers and unbelievers. The intent is not to answer the specific issues in detail but to provide New and Old Testament frameworks from which elder care can be viewed relative to the family.

Sadly, at some level, every family is dysfunctional due to our human nature. Some, of course, are more so than others. The deepest dysfunctions can occur with abuse and neglect. The Bible speaks clearly about the ill-treatment of others, particularly when the recipient is defenseless. Abuse and neglect are not only wrong but also criminal. If you suspect abuse or neglect of physical, emotional, or financial nature, contact law enforcement, adult protective services, or an agency serving elders. Even if unsubstantiated, the defenseless need protection.

Family relationships can be difficult. They become more challenging to negotiate during a time of crisis. In families with relational issues, it can be helpful to speak together as a family before anything happens to an elder. Members can discuss "what if" scenarios.

"What if something should happen? How should we respond?" If family members have a history of conflict, sometimes a "truce" can be called. While recognizing a relational problem, the elder's crisis trumps the individual's problem. The focus is on the elder's care and the decisions that need to be made. There is no easy way around the sticky family issues, though a humble approach to working toward the benefit of the elder is helpful. Remember, it is hard to argue with a humble person.

Facing issues of an aging family member or friend, or our own aging, is something most people try to avoid. Yet it is much easier to face with having discussions early on, a realistic appraisal of the situation, reaching out for support and information, and keeping Philippians 2:3–4 in mind: "Do nothing out of selfish ambition or vain conceit. Rather, in humility value others above yourselves, not looking to your own interests but each of you to the interests of others."

Approaching Our Own Aging: Retirement

As we consider the Scriptures, we can see that God designed us to age. Though God's original plan for us was corrupted by sin (though we shall rise to the incorruptible), our bodies are self-healing and "wonderfully made" (Ps. 139:14), a blessing from God. Though we are subject to disease from within and without, most of the time our bodies heal themselves and work in mysterious ways—from conception, through life, and until we die. The reality is that we do not fall ill as much as we could because of the implicit defenses our bodies have to ward off diseases, germs, viruses, and infections.

In the garden of Eden, speaking to the man and woman before the corruption of sin, "God blessed them and said to them, 'Be fruitful and increase in number; fill the earth and subdue it. Rule over the fish in the sea and the birds in the sky and over every living creature that moves on the ground'" (Gen. 1:28). He says in verse 29 that seed-bearing plants and animals of the field are to provide food for them. God is providing the food, but the man and woman need to gather and prepare it to eat. God is blessing them with two things: provisions and work. Both are blessed before the great corruption.

After the corruption, God speaks to Adam and Eve in Genesis 3 of curses that increase the pain of childbirth, hard and painful toil to produce food, the introduction of thistles and thorns to make growing and harvesting more difficult, and the return of their bodies todeath. Pain, toil, sweat, thorns, hardship, and death brought to us courtesy of the corruption. God will reverse this as he carries out his ultimate plan, but until then life is hard. And work is hard, fraught with challenges and problems whether we toil in the literal or figurative fields.

Years of hard work lead us to look forward to retirement, right? But the concept of retirement is not found in the Scriptures. In 1935, the US Social Security System set the retirement age at sixty-five. While not entirely clear as to why that age was chosen, several US business and state pension plans at the time used sixty-five, while the US Railroad Pension was sixty-four. An actuarial study was done at the time, and it was believed that a modest payroll tax would make the Social Security System self-sustaining.[1] From a pragmatic perspective, sixty-five was reasonable at that time. Life expectancy of those who live to that age has seen a modest increase since the 1930s. A gradual increase in the "full retirement" age was implemented to possibly ensure the program's stability and to continue to make actuarial sense.

If work is a blessing from God—and it makes sense that it is how we "produce food" and shelter for ourselves and families—should we stop working at our full retirement age? We never really do stop working in the sense that food needs to be gathered and prepared and shelter maintained through the balance of life. The only difference is the source of payment while we continue to live.

An increased percentage of people die in the few years after retirement. However, the data analysts for and against early retirement have mixed reviews regarding if early retirement adds to years or detracts. The time to leave the workforce is an individual question based on personal status and other factors, all of which are not the purpose of this writing. The point here is whether retirement is "from" or "to." God has blessed us with work. We can certainly choose to retire to a life of leisure, but the data suggest that work keeps us involved with other people (social engagement), provides more active day-to-day life, and employs our brains. These all contribute to a meaningful life.

We do not retire from ourselves or life itself. It is better to consider retirement not so much as going from work as retiring to something meaningful that can be done in this next phase of life. Some men retire to play golf. After a time, golf can become less absorbing and fun if it is all a retiree is doing. Other people retire from the corporate world to use their talents and experience in helping non-profit ministries, teaching, or mentoring. It is better to look forward to something than just saying good riddance to a job. Not being responsible for work that is not enjoyable is a relief but does not meet our social and emotional needs for what is next in life.

Experiencing the Gifts of Aging

God does bless the aging. Clearly, he loves and cares for the aging, and he reserves special gifts that typically come as we age.

People sometimes say they wish they had had grandchildren before their children. Why? Grandchildren bring joy and wonder to life in a way few other things can. As we age, we have more time and different priorities and perspectives than when we were raising our families. The pressures of careers and debts may have reduced over the years, and we can enjoy the simple pleasure of being with a grandchild.

Grandchildren benefit from the attention and love of grandparents, even when they are not able to be together often. The more the grandparent makes efforts to connect with the grandchildren, the deeper that relationship impacts the grandchildren for life. Many people who work with the aging will point to a key grandparent in their lives as to why they love working with older people. We went into this in more detail in chapter 3, so suffice it to say that grandchildren are a blessing that comes only with years of experience and can be a top gift of aging.

Experience comes only with age. When combined with wisdom, experience can be a powerful blessing. For example, once you learn how certain cons or scams work, the less likely you fall prey to them. But the advice and insight you learn from even the bad experiences can be a great help to others. From a long-term perspective, we learn about decisions and choices in life that simply do not work or can take us down unwise paths. Experience teaches us the value of friends, that money does not create happiness, that love can come at any age, and so many more truths. When the woman caught in adultery was brought before Jesus to trap him, his response was, "He who is without sin should cast the first stone." The older men turned and left first. They quickly recognized their sin and that they could not qualify as sinless. It took the younger men longer to realize this before they, too, left. Why? They had not had the life experience of the older men.

Experience combined with wisdom can cause a profound effect. As discussed earlier, the use of wisdom in the Hebrew sense is skill in living. Experience may teach us that a child is making a bad decision. Wisdom helps us know how to communicate it to the child. In management, some vital aphorisms new managers should pay attention to include "It's not what you say, but how you say it" and "They may forget what you said, but they will never forget how you made them feel." Those statements were born of experience and wisdom.

Years ago, when I was still in my twenties, the nursing center I administered was offered an adjacent property to purchase. In talking over the offer, an old farmer told me, "The time to buy is when it's for sale." Proverbs teach wisdom that comes from the experience of the writer; a good portion came from King Solomon, the man on whom God bestowed wisdom. Proverbs are to teach the young, but they also inform the aging. Skill in living comes after years of success and failure in living. The wise listen to good counsel and learn from experience. Experience combined with wisdom is a trait that comes through listening and applying the Bible to daily life and observing how the Word provides insight.

Not long ago three friends and I had a reunion of sorts. The four of us had not been together in the same room for forty years. Two of the guys' wives that we all knew from college were able to come along as well. When we met one another for the first time after all those years, we clung together in a group hug. As we stood in the parking lot, arms locked, one of the wives began singing a song we had all learned in college where we had met. The moment was unforgettable and precious, one I still think of fondly. Friends we have known and loved for years, even if separated for a time, seem to pick up where they left off. Shared memories and comfort and trust with an old friend is unlike any other experience. Friends like these are a gift only the aging can understand. I know of two college roommates from the early 1970s who served together on nonprofit boards and still go on vacations together. They can have differences, but their memories and years together create a safe binding around them, and they go on together. David and Jonathon had a relationship closer than brothers that lasted long after Jonathon died. David searched for Jonathon's remaining family members and found one, Mephibosheth, who ate at David's table for his remaining days.

Sometimes family members carry the attributes of good friends. The brothers and sisters who are also good friends are a gift upon gift. Not only are they friends but also have a shared life from the earliest days. They know one another's roots and the foibles and lore of the family. Secrets shared as children are often still held, only to come out at just the right time or kept forever sealed. A sibling-friend does not happen often, but those who have it are truly blessed.

Seeing children and grandchildren grow and mature can be exciting, scary, and affirming in many ways. To have them also express faith in Jesus is not guaranteed to any home. To receive that gift brings joy and comfort that only serving together a beloved Father can. It allows parents and their adult children to share in a faith life that mutually encourages and sustains in both hard times and good. A son and daughter who walk with honor before the Lord is a wonderful thing to see. A blessing shared in Psalm 128:6 is "May you live to see your children's children—peace be on Israel." Just to see grandchildren brings joy, and when they come from generations serving the Lord, it is an increased blessing.

Not all of these blessings are shared by everyone. Some of us experience the exact opposite of the blessing. But there is a blessing for that situation as well. The Lord never sleeps or slumbers, and his words never return to him without having the effect he sent them out with. The lessons and prayers over your children may seem lost to them as they age, but they remain inside of them. God is not done loving them and drawing them to him, and he continues to call them to him. It is wise not to judge too harshly or early for something that God has not yet finished. As Paul said in 1 Corinthians 13, "There remain these three things—faith, hope, and love, and the greatest of these is love." With these three we can continue living in hope, the knowledge that God loves us and has a future for us that remains even as we age. This, too, is a blessing. "Whoever dwells in the shelter of the Most High Will rest in the shadow of the Almighty" (Ps. 91:1).

One final blessing that God gives us is one we can use at all ages but gets the most use as we age. That is the gift of knowing that there is a hope in the future. This is not the future of our children or of meaningful activities to come. It is the future after we give up this life. Regardless of how bad our experiences and how deep our losses during life, God promises to dry every tear and fill our every need. We are held closely in his hands and heart, and he refuses to let us go. We cannot escape from him, nor will he ever reject us. Paul says in Romans 8:39, "Neither height nor depth, nor anything else in all creation, will be able to separate us from the love of God that is in Christ Jesus our Lord." He is the author and perfector of our faith and the one true hope we have in this life. But there is more.

This same hope that is in us in Christ is in others who trust in him too. It is for all who revere Christ in their hearts. That means that anyone who loves the Lord and passes away before we do are neither gone nor forgotten. They are hidden in Christ from our view now. The reality is that we will see them later. For believers, every goodbye, even at the grave, is "See you later." This statement is not to decry the pain we feel when a loved one passes on. The grief is real. So is the future reality. It does not take away the loss; it removes some of death's sting. Why? Because of hope. Hope gives strength and knowledge, that even in loss, all is not lost. Because of Jesus.

> Praise the Lord, my soul;
> All my inmost being, praise his holy name.
> Praise the Lord my soul, and forget not his
> benefits—
> Who forgives all your sins
> And heals all your diseases,
> Who redeems your life from the pit
> And crowns you with love and compassion.
> Who satisfies your desires with good things
> So that your youth is renewed like the eagle's.
> (Ps. 103:1–5)

Application

I wonder what Adam felt when God first said his name. He had to look at God and nature surrounding him and marvel at how he, too, was God's creation. The psalmist wrote, "I am fearfully and wonderfully made…Marvelous are thy works!" We are the epitome of God's creative conscience and energy. Implicit within this body of ours is the design for years of living and growing. We are made in the image of God, and that fact alone is sufficient for praising God. Then considering how we are designed to self-heal, grow, and replicate is a miracle, but how we age is a marvel in and of itself. Being made in God's image and the wonder of how our bodies function and age are all reasons to respect one another, especially elders. God tells us that the aged deserve our highest regard because he made them and for the years of life he graced them.

We are told to respect elders, and God provided us examples of how to respect and love them through the law, history, poetry, and prophets of the Bible. Jesus himself showed respect for elders. Was calling the Pharisees a "brood of vipers" and "blind guides" an act of respect? He could have caused the buildings to fall on them or hit them with selective lighting or even curse them, but he did not. That was respect, if not for the Pharisees then for the people God loves and created.

In rehab programs for alcoholics, the persons who love the alcoholics but have been hurt by them sometimes stage an "intervention" to confront the alcoholic loved ones. The purpose is twofold. First, they need to vent their pain. Second, alcoholics need to hear the truth of their disease. It is direct, intense, and painful for the receiver of those words. Only by hearing the direct truth in the strongest possible words can the addicted person begin to accept the reality of his disease. When someone loves a person who refuses to listen, often strong, honest rebuking is required to make him or her think. The Pharisees were not addicted to alcohol; rather, they were addicted to their self-righteousness and delusion by lies. Jesus used strong, bracing language because they refused to heed his call to recognize the truth before them. If God is love and Jesus is love, Jesus did not hate the Pharisees. Confronting them was the last chance he had before his death to verbally shake them saying, "Listen to me! Look in the Scriptures and see the truth!" We are to respect and love all by the power of God's Holy Spirit, even when sometimes we must confront in love.

Honest, intense love can be the backdrop for all our family interactions from this day forward. It is seen in Jesus, our perfect Advocate, how he exhibited all aspects of God's goodness, even when calling people to task. Speaking the truth in love is one way God helps us to serve those who are sometimes hard to love. Knowing that we speak truth to people we love will later give comfort, though they may oppose our thinking now. During those long, difficult days, never forget that when we are serving elders and the needy, however humble the task, we are serving the beloved of God.

Paul wrote in 1 Corinthians that love bears all things and never gives up. When siblings or our elders refuse to recognize or deal with the circumstances, we can either give up or work to keep an open dialogue. Elders will sometimes make decisions that are contrary to what we think is best, and that is their prerogative as adults. At times we may have to allow elders to live through the consequences of those contrary decisions and be ready to catch them later, and the only way to do that is to continue nourishing the relationship with them. We can be direct about our feelings and still support one another.

Like when Jim let his mom continue to drive the half-mile to the church and store after she vehemently refused to give up her car keys. She was so adamant that she used words Jim did not think she knew! Her life revolved around her church, friends at church, and going to the grocery store. She refused to let anyone take away her independence and joy those times gave her. In the following two years, she had no accidents and no injuries, but she relinquished her keys voluntarily. In her own time, she decided when to give up driving. Walking was getting difficult, and her best friends at church had died. So long as safety is maintained, giving older people time to adjust and make the right decisions is a way we may lose a battle but win the war.

We can change our perspectives of aging in how God made us and in recognizing the various gifts aging people receive. Someone said the gift of aging is having grandchildren during the day then giving them back at the day's end. Grandchildren are wonderful but are not God's only gift as people age. In our relationships with elders, we can look for and encourage the expression of the gifts of aging in those we love.

As we recognize elders' deepening love for God as well as their legacy, courage, frankness, and so on, we are affirming the value of the elders' years and what we can learn from them. In this we find that they are far more valuable than their earthly possessions. Whether they possess many assets or few, they remain great in our eyes, a blessing for us for the remainder of our years. In recognizing God's gifts bestowed on and through them, they can live in dignity.

Takeaway Thoughts

My intention with this book is to help you see how God values each of us as we and those around us grow older. While he cannot love us more than he already does, older people are precious in his sight. When we read and understand how deeply God feels toward us throughout life and continues to bless us through the years, we can see greater value in our relationship with him. Has this book changed your perspective of how God sees your aging? How about your perspective of the aging of the elders and family in your life?

A person read an early version of this manuscript, and it caused her to reflect on the years of her relationship with her mother. Have you been rethinking your parent and sibling relationships as you considered this material? Do you think any part of your prior relationships with parents and siblings would have been different had you thought through them as the Scriptures suggest? How can you take what you have thought about God's viewpoint and use it to benefit the elders in your life? Has this material changed how you pray for your loved ones?

We all make mistakes in our relationships with elders and family members. This book does not highlight any failures in our caring for elders; rather, we are focusing on how we use failures as springboards to redevelop relationships and honor the aged by God's powerful grace and to give him glory.

Questions for Consideration

1. Given all we have discussed throughout this book, what is the significance of Scripture recording the advanced ages of many people when they started their most effective ministries? For example, Abraham, Jacob, Moses, Aaron, and others.

2. In what ways has your view of aging changed through this reading book?

3. What gifts do you think you would most like to develop that come through aging?

4. How do you think comorbidity will affect the ones you love? Yourself? What can you do today to reduce the impact of comorbidity in your elders' lives and yourself?

5. How do you view your retirement planning? How does it relate to your faith? How do you think that receiving an estate will affect you or your fellow beneficiaries' relation-

ships? How will giving an estate affect you or your heirs' relationships?

6. Are you aware of someone's guilt for placing a parent in an institution for their care? How could you respond to that person? If you are feeling guilty because you had to make the hard decision to place your parent in an institution for care, how can your faith and trust in Christ help you?

7. How have you become more thoughtful and aware of aging and how that process is addressed in Scripture?

8. How do you feel about the "See you later" rather than the "Goodbye" perspective?

RESOURCES

The following resources are provided for your information and further research:

Abuse and Exploitation and Elder Justice Initiative

    Specific information from the US Department of Justice related to victims of elder abuse and financial exploitation and their families: https://www.justice.gov/elderjustice.

    National Center for Elder Abuse provides resources on elder abuse prevention, including information on reporting a suspected case of elder abuse: https://ncea.acl.gov/.

    National Adult Protective Services Association provides a map to locate the closest Adult Protective Services for victims of physical abuse and/or financial exploitation: http://www.napsa-now.org/get-help/help-in-your-area/.

    Find helpful resources to prevent and respond to elder abuse: https://www.elderjustice.gov.

Administration on Aging (AoA)

    This comprehensive website provides information for older adults, family caregivers, and professionals. It includes a Resource Directory for Older People and information on using the Eldercare Locator, a national toll-free, directory-assistance service designed to help older persons and their caregivers locate support services in their local areas: www.aoa.gov.

Administration for Community Living

This site contains a wide array of information on programs for older adults and persons with disabilities: https://www.acl.gov/, 202-619-0724,

Aging and Care Services

Information about care and services from nonprofit providers of aging services: LeadingAge.org.

Aging Information (General Family)

A search for aging information on the Focus on the Family website provides good material relating to family issues and life with aging parents: focusonthefamily.com.

Aging Services Directory

The Senate Committee on Aging website provides an excellent variety of relevant information for seniors and those who care for them: www.aging.senate.gov.
National Institute on Aging provides aging-related health information easily assessable for adults sixty and over: https://www.nia.nih.gov/health.

Alzheimer's Disease and Dementia

The Alzheimer's Association is a leading voluntary health organization in Alzheimer's care, support, and research: www.alz.org.
National Institute on Aging website provides current, comprehensive, and unbiased information about Alzheimer's disease: https://www.nia.nih.gov/health/alzheimers or Alzheimers.gov, 800-438-4380.
American Association of Retired Persons (AARP): AARP.org.

Consumer Financial Protection Bureau provides easy-to-understand guides to help financial caregivers managing someone else's money: https://www.consumerfinance.gov/consumer-tools/managing-someone-elses-money/.

Do-Not-Call Complaints

The National Do-Not-Call Complaints online form and telephone number are available if you are registered with National Do-Not-Call Registry and you receive an unsolicited telemarketing call: https://consumercomplaints.fcc.gov/hc/en-us, 1-888-CALL-FCC (1-888-225-5322) / TTY: 1-888-835-5322.

Information about the National Do-Not-Call Registry, which can stop telemarketers from calling your home or mobile phone is available at https://www.donotcall.gov/.

Federal Communications Commission provides information on what to do when receiving an unsolicited call from an individual you suspect is not being honest about who they are or where they are calling from https://consumercomplaints.fcc.gov/hc/en-us.

Elder Care

Everything families need to understand, plan, and manage care for their elderly loved ones through the caregiving years is available at the Care Guide: www.careguide.com.

Aging parents: 8 warning signs of health problems. Use this guide to gauge how your aging parents are doing—and what to do if they need help: https://www.mayoclinic.org/healthy-lifestyle/caregivers/in-depth/aging-parents/art-20044126.

Aging parents: Signs it's time to step in—and the best ways to help. Lauren Levy, 12/30/2020. This and similar articles identify what "red flags" to look for that might indicate an elder needs more help. https://www.care.com/c/stories/5412/9-signs-your-parent-needs-help/.

Eldercare Locator

National Administration on Aging offers a nationwide toll-free service to help find community assistance for seniors: eldercare.acl. gov, 800-677-1116.

National Center on Caregiving provides information on caring for family members with chronic illness or disability: www.caregiver. org.

National Association of Area Agencies on Aging is a federal agency with connections to local Area Agencies on Aging: https:// www.n4a.org/.

Energy Assistance

Low Income Home Energy Assistance Program website contains general information on the Low Income Home Energy Assistance Program (LIHEAP): https://www.acf.hhs.gov/ocs/programs/liheap.

Exercise and Activity

National Institute on Aging's program Go4Life is an exercise and physical activity campaign designed to help adults fifty and over to put exercise and physical activity into their daily lives: https:// go4life.nia.nih.gov/.

Financial Information

Aging Care provides news and information about financial issues important to seniors: Agingcare.com.

Money Smart for Older Adults provides awareness among older adults and their caregivers on how to prevent elder financial exploitation and encourages advance planning and informed financial decision-making: https://files.consumerfinance.gov/f/201306_cfpb_msoa-partici-pant-guide.pdf.

American Association of Daily Money Managers helps find financial professionals who provide personal financial/bookkeeping services to senior citizens and the disabled: https://secure.aadmm. com.

Healthy Aging

Centers for Disease Control and Prevention's site provides a variety of information relating to seniors' life, health, and safety: http://www.cdc.gov/aging/.

The CDC has excellent resources for assessing and reducing falls: https://www.cdc.gov/features/falls-older-adults/index.html.

Healthfinder supplies links to selected online publications, clearinghouses, databases, websites, and support and self-help groups, as well as government agencies and nonprofit organizations for seniors and others: https://healthfinder.gov/.

Staying Healthy and aging well website publishes a guide providing tips to help prepare and cope with the changes that go with growing older—and live life to the fullest. https://www.helpguide. org/articles/alzheimers-dementia-aging/staying-healthy-as-you-age. htm.

Housing

Information related to housing options for seniors including HUD housing programs: https://portal.hud.gov/hudportal/ HUD?src=/topics/information_for_senior_citizens.

HUD Supportive Housing for the Elderly Program information about the Section 202 program is helping to expand the supply of affordable housing with supportive services for the elderly: https:// www.hud.gov.

Find out if you are eligible for a mortgage modification or refinancing: Making Home Affordable.gov, 1-888-995-HOPE (4673).

Nursing Home Compare is a Medicare site that provides detailed information about the past performance of every Medicare and Medicaid certified nursing home in the country: https://www. medicare.gov/nursinghomecompare/search.html?.

Hospice

Information regarding medical care to help someone with a terminal illness live as well as possible for as long as possible, increasing quality of life, is found at: https://hospicefoundation.org/Hospice-Care/Hospice-Services.

Identity Theft

Federal Trade Commission, Identity Theft Resource Center, has resources to help protect people from identity theft. The nonprofit organization provides victim assistance to consumers throughout the United States, at no charge: https://www.consumer.ftc.gov/features/feature-0014-identity-theft.

Legal Assistance

The National Academy of Elder Law Attorneys is a directory of elder and special needs law attorneys with experience working on behalf of seniors: https://www.naela.org.

Medicare Information

The Official US Government Site for People with Medicare: https://www.medicare.gov/.

Medicaid

The federal website provides information about medical assistance for certain low-income families: www.medicaid.gov.

Medication Tips for Seniors

The Food and Drug Administration has numerous publications with information for older people on medication use and safety:

REVEALING GOD'S DESIGN FOR AGING, FAMILY,
AND HOW WE LIVE

https://www.fda.gov/drugs/drug-information-consumers/tips-se-niors, 1-888-INFO-FDA (1-888-463-6332).

Nutrition

A federal resource that provides access to online federal government information on nutrition is found at: https://www.nutrition.gov.

Scam Information

The Better Business Bureau Scam Tracker provides resources and information exposing fraudulent schemes: https://www.bbb.org/scamtracker.

Senior Living has a comprehensive guide examining common scams that target older Americans: seniorliving.org.

Senior Living

Developed by the private sector, Senior Living provides information on eldercare and long-term care. Senior Living provides numerous links to information on legal, financial, medical, and housing issues, as well as policy, research, and statistics: www.seniorliving.org.

Social Security Administration

The Social Security Administration toll-free number operates from 7:00 AM to 7:00 PM, Monday through Friday. Recorded information and services are available twenty-four hours a day. The website contains a wealth of information and resources: https://www.ssa.gov/, 800-772-1213.

Spouse Support

The Well Spouse Foundation gives support information to partners of the chronically ill/disabled: www.wellspouse.org/.

Veterans

The Guide to Long-Term Care for Veterans provides information about long-term care options for Veterans—home and community-based, and residential care: https://www.va.gov/GERIATRICS/Guide/LongTermCare/index.asp.

Volunteer Opportunities

Created for people fifty-five and older, the Senior Corps has three components: Foster Grandparents, Senior Companions, and Retired and Senior Volunteers (RSVP): https://www.nationalservice.gov/programs/senior-corps, 1-800-424-8867.

AUTHOR'S NOTE AND ACKNOWLEDGMENTS

Few meaningful endeavors are successful through the effort of one person alone. Certainly, there are leaders and prime movers in projects and events, but they alone are in the visible eye, some by choice and others by chance.

This work is the result of the encouragement, challenge, and insight of others. The story behind the story is that in 2013, the leader of an Adult Bible Fellowship of Hope Church in Mason, Ohio, requested a brief presentation on the dynamics people in the group were experiencing with their aging parents. The result was the creation of a five-week series on how the Scriptures speak about aging and the aged and how that perspective can inform the relationships with elders in our lives. The group's response underscored a need to examine the Bible's insights on how to live well through the issues of aging within the family. I am grateful to the people of Hope Church who encouraged and informed me on what they needed to hear.

A year after the sessions were over, the book idea began with a few chapters. My wife and some friends read the material and encouraged me to continue. Then I took a new job in another state, and the book completely stalled out for seven years. During a conference at the Cove in Ashville, North Carolina, a "chance" meeting with Dr. Larry Crabb occurred. We spoke only briefly but somehow landed on the scriptural aspects of aging. Frankly, I cannot say exactly what he said, but what I heard was something like "I'd like to read about that." Sometimes single comments can redirect our trajectory. His words (or whatever he actually said!) deeply spurred me to again pick up and continue with the manuscript.

The completion of this book would not have occurred without the guidance and encouragement of my sister, Betty, and many friends. Paul Tedder and the Monday Morning Men's Bible Study, both of Fellowship Greenville, were gracious with their insight and suggestions. Erin Brown worked tirelessly on multiple edits, teaching me how to think and write better. I am grateful for her viewpoint, ideas, and recommendations. I am indebted to Nina, my wife, whose patient listening, reading, and giving up together-time not only supported this work but was essential. Thank you, all.

Finally, any errors are solely mine; any truth is singularly God's.